ASSESSING HEALTH CARE

a study in
organisational evaluation

Gilbert Smith and Caroline Cantley

Open University Press

Milton Keynes · Philadelphia

Open University Press
12 Cofferidge Close
Stony Stratford
Milton Keynes MK11 1BY, England
and
242 Cherry Street
Philadelphia, PA 19106, USA

First Published 1985

British Library Cataloguing in Publication Data

Smith, Gilbert
Assessing health care: a study in organizational evaluation.
1. Daycare hospitals for the aged - Great Britain - Evaluation
I. Title II. Cantley, Caroline
362.6'1 HV1481.G53

ISBN 0-335-15072-1

Library of Congress Cataloging in Publication Data

Smith, Gilbert A., 1944-
Assessing health care.

Bibliography: p.
Includes index.
1. Hospital care—Evaluation. 2. Aged—Hospital care—Evaluation—Case studies. I. Cantley, Caroline. II. Title.
RA972.S65 1985 362.1'1 84-27215

ISBN 0-335-15072-1

Text Design by Nicola Sheldon

Typeset by
Butler & Tanner Ltd, Frome and London
Printed in Great Britain by
Thomson Litho Ltd, East Kilbride, Scotland

Contents

Acknowledgements

A research project of this kind is only completed with a great deal of help from other people.

Professor Raymond Illsley first suggested the project. The Scottish Home and Health Department (SHHD) provided grant support. Professor F.M. Martin, as head of the Department of Social Administration and Social Work at the University of Glasgow, where the research was initially based, gave much assistance and encouragement.

Valeria Ritman was a member of the research team and helped with data collection from January 1981 until she left the project in the autumn of 1982.

Helen Dalrymple was our research secretary in Glasgow, with help from May Miller and Carol Brown. When the project moved to the University of Hull, Sue Needham added much work on the research (including preparing the final typescript) to her duties as a departmental secretary. We are particularly grateful to her.

A number of colleagues have commented on working papers or chapters in draft. We thank Andy Alaszewski, Robert Chester, David Hunter, Douglas Hooper, David May, Stuart Montgomery, David Robinson and Chris Walker who also advised us on word processing. Chapter 5 draws on an article that was published in *Ageing and Society* (Smith and Cantley with Ritman 1983) and Chapter 10 is a much expanded version of a research note which appeared in *The British Journal of Social Work* (Cantley and Smith 1983).

Finally we are very grateful to those who co-operated with us on the research but who, for reasons of research confidentiality, must remain anonymous; the members and officials of the relevant Health Board, the consultant and staff at the day hospital, which we studied, and (above all others) the patients and their relatives.

CHAPTER ONE

Directions in Evaluative Research

Introduction

Whatever the stated objectives of research on health and welfare services, one issue is of particular significance. That is the issue of evaluation. Certainly, most social scientific investigations of these services have a significant evaluative component, either built into them, or subsequently imposed upon their results by those who have an interest in using research for evaluative purposes. Interest in evaluation is particularly strong where the service under investigation is an innovative one, although this concern is present also in research on established forms of service provision.

Because of the prevalence of interest in evaluating health and welfare, a clear formulation of the research question and a sound research strategy to provide the answer are very important. This importance has been well recognized and a voluminous literature on the methodology of evaluative research, over a considerable period of time (Hyman and Wright 1968; Schwartz and Alwin 1971; Goldberg and Connelly, eds. 1981; Goldberg 1984), speaks to the point. Yet, in spite of this attention, a satisfactory methodological approach has proved surprisingly elusive. The execution of evaluative research still has major problems. As Weiss (1972, pp. 24–25) has explained:

> The evaluation question sounds simple enough in the abstract ... But what looks elementary in theory turns out in practice to be a demanding enterprise. Programs are nowhere near as neat and accommodating as the evaluator expects. Nor are outside circumstances as passive and unimportant as he might like. Whole platoons of unexpected problems spring up.

And in spite of the persistent nature of these problems there is little evidence that solutions have yet been advanced that command widespread support amongst social scientists. Goldberg and Connelly (1981, p. 313) can only conclude an extensive collection of reports, in *Evaluative Research in Social Care*, with the comment that:

> The heated discussions of the pros and cons of the use of different methodologies in evaluating outcomes seemed to signify a search for the most relevant approach according to the state of theoretical knowledge, the state of the art of intervention techniques, and the constraints of the field setting. There was agreement that evaluation of social care demands many different approaches.

This seems to be a polite way of saying that evaluation research is still in a state of considerable disarray. Certainly as we embarked upon a study designed initially to assess the efficacy of a new health service, we rapidly became dissatisfied with the approaches which were available to guide us.

So the issue of evaluation is at the heart of this book. That is why, although the volume is primarily a report on our research, we begin with an overview of the approaches that have been taken in assessing health and welfare care. We shall argue that major problems have arisen and have persisted because some of the presumptions about social policy, social research and organizations, which underlie many evaluations, are unjustified. In consequence a mode of evaluative research has evolved – essentially experimental, rationalist and objectivist in approach – which is fraught with difficulty. We shall suggest an alternative mode. Our report in the body of the book seeks to demonstrate the advantages of this alternative; advantages which we summarize and set out explicitly in the final chapter. The data which we report and which were collected in a new psychogeriatric day hospital are thus presented as a general demonstration of the way in which evaluation may proceed in a wide range of health and welfare services. Throughout the book our central argument is that there are significant gains to be made by departing from an essentially rationalist and experimental approach and moving towards a more pluralistic stance.

Some problems

We begin with the observation that there are major problems with evaluative research which have their origins in methodological weaknesses.

The first problem is that empirical research results have not had the impact upon professional practice and upon social policy that they might have had. Garland et al. (1981) argue for a reassessment of the role of evaluation research in, for example, planning for alternatives to institutional care for the elderly. He feels that the major methodological weaknesses of many evaluative studies have meant that research has not influenced policies for long-term care. He rejects research designed to perfect some ideal model of care. Rather he favours studies which will improve the information available to clients, families and service providers, thus allowing *them* to establish *their* preferences. In the same field of service provision Kelman (1980) has developed the point. He has little doubt that strategies of evaluation in studies of health services for the elderly are underdeveloped. He highlights methodological problems in the use of controls, in coping with the 'flexible' nature of the programme being evaluated, and in establishing that any one set of measures of input can be validly held to be the criteria of the programmes objectives.

Of course methodological weakness is not the only barrier to an effective relationship between research on the one hand and policy and practice on the other. Cherns et al. (1972), Crawford and Perry (1976), Bulmer (1982) and Gandy et al. (eds. 1983) have all demonstrated that this relationship is very complicated. Nevertheless, as Robertson and Gandy (1983, p. 246) argue, there are good grounds for pointing to the limitations of the currently predominant approach to evaluation as one of the more important reasons for the apparent lack of influence of research upon policy. The design of many evaluations means that:

> They are unable to specify with any precision which, and to what extent, particular factors within the policy, treatment-method or regime, etc. assessed by the research have contributed to the results (normally defined in terms of the stated 'objectives' of the programme under scrutiny) the programme has achieved.

Thus it may be difficult to assess whether a programme's achievements are attributable to its content or to some other factors. This failing is crucial since the whole point of most evaluations is to 'attempt to assess the effects produced by policies or programmes, and the extent to which such results measure up to programme "goals" (however these may be defined)' (p. 246).

So, much policy research is essentially evaluative, the quality of design in evaluative research is therefore important and yet, typically, conventional designs are beset with problems. Now we detail these problems more fully and suggest why they have occurred.

Most often the description of an evaluative design runs like this: define service goals, specify service outcomes as measures of goal achievement, define criteria of success, isolate the effects of the service from other possible causes, measure achievements, and adjudicate on the success (or otherwise) of the service. Of course, it could be argued that this is an oversimplified statement of traditional evaluation, presented so as to render it amenable to easy criticism. The fact is, however, that there is a remarkable degree of agreement amongst commentators as to the key features of mainstream evaluative research. Compare, for instance, Bulmer (1982, p. 159):

> Evaluation research typically has a five-stage structure. (a) Find out the goals of the (limited) policy being evaluated; (b) translate the goals into measurable indicators of goal achievement; (c) collect data on these indicators for the study participants who have been exposed to the programme; (d) collect similar data on an equivalent group that has not been exposed to the programme; (e) compare the results for the experimental and control groups in relation to the goals set.

and Illsley (1980, p. 113):

> The classic evaluative model . . . has several distinctive features. These are:
> 1. The primary objective of the intervention can be unequivocally specified.
> 2. It tests the effectiveness and/or efficiency of a given product or process in achieving the goal compared with alternative interventions or with no intervention.

3. It has a precise, foreseeable and measurable control over the nature and quality of the input.
4. Influences extraneous to the measured input, the controlled intervention process, and the measured output can be excluded by research design.
5. The criterion of success is uncontroversial and can be measured on a single dimension.

Goldberg and Connelly (1982), too, stress throughout their thorough review of recent and current evaluative research, especially in the context of services for the elderly, that: 'The evaluative process starts with the identification of aims, goes on to the definition and assessment of needs, the descriptions and monitoring of input and moves finally to the measurement of outcome.' (p. 37)

The difficulty is that the approach to evaluation reflected in these statements rests upon three presumptions – about the 'policy process' (Hill, 1983), about social research and about organizations – which are frequently unjustified. We term these the presumption of rationality in social policy, the presumption of the experimental ideal in social research and the presumption of consensus in professional organizations.

The presumption of rationality

The first presumption that is often made is the presumption of rationality. Carley (1980, p. 10) defines rationality in a policy context as follows:

> ... in economic thought, to be rational is to select from a group of alternative courses of action that course which maximizes output for a given input, or minimizes input for a given output ... in systems analysis, decision theory, or game theory, to be rational is to select a course of action, from a group of possible courses of action which has a given set of predicted consequences, in terms of some welfare function which, in turn, ranks each set of consequences in order of preference.

As Carley further explains, 'rational man' proceeds to make and implement policy through a series of sequentially linked activities which closely parallel the stages of evaluation that we have already described. In summary, (1) a problem is identified and goals and values organized; (2) all solutions are listed; (3) consequences are predicted; (4) consequences are compared, and (5) a strategy is selected on the basis of costs and benefits. If we presume that the policy process is rational in these terms, then all is well for traditional evaluation. There is a 'fit' between the mode of evaluation and the presumed character of that which is being evaluated. As Hyman and Wright (1968, p. 742) note, 'Evaluation has come to be accepted, even sought, as an accompaniment to rational action.'

Problems arise, however, because we now know that this representation of the policy process is generally inaccurate. It is merely an ideal model. Carley adds (p. 11):

> It is worth stresing for the first of many times that these steps constitute an ideal model ... A model ... is not reality. In so far as this rational model diverges from reality in its attempts at simplification it is bound to be open to criticism, and there is indeed a considerable body of critical literature.

Smith and May (1980) have summarized the debate. The rationalistic approach is too narrow in neglecting a range of significant political variables, especially the power of relevant vested interests. The approach (as we have noted) is utopian. The conditions under which it applies are exceptional. It is value-biased in that rationality tends to be equated with the smooth running of the organization and is therefore itself a value generally favouring senior management and other 'top dogs'. The distinction that is drawn between ends and means, or goals and strategies, is too rigid. It has even been suggested that the ideal rational model is, in any case, impractical largely because of the high costs of making decisions in a rational way.

In the present context we are most concerned with those aspects of these criticisms which are of direct relevance to evaluative research. There are four points. First, the rational model is an *ideal*. In practice, policy making is very confused. Evaluations must reflect that. House (1980, p. 19) explains:

> The actual evaluative process is more complicated than it would appear. People evaluate not only by applying standards but also by checking their judgements against particular situations in which they feel confident that they know the outcome. Actual evaluative reasoning proceeds more as a dialectical process between abstract principles and concrete example than as straightforward deduction from standards.

Second, the rational model points to clear goals. That, too, is unreal. Rather, ambiguity and confusion of purpose are *typical* and not at all unusual features of most agencies. A good deal of research in hospitals and other organizations (Strauss et al. 1964; Eldridge and Crombie 1974; Silverman 1979) has shown that objectives vary between and within significant groups. Goals of services are complex, multiple, conflicting and vary over time and between contexts. They are variously interpreted, notoriously ambiguous, and are sometimes difficult to locate at all. As Cronbach et al. (1980, p. 129) add:

> References to the attainment of goals pervade discussion of social programs and their evaluation ... but this [point of view] seems rationalist to the point of unreality. Consensus on ends and priorities is mostly absent from a context of accommodation.
>
> For rationalists, all thinking starts with a specified goal or purpose. To find a means to the stated end is what it means to 'solve a problem', *but that is not how social action is taken.* [italics added]

Martin Rein (1976) reinforces the point. In describing his own approach to the analysis of social policy he advances a curt rubric: treat the question of purpose as unresolved. He explains (p. 21): 'In analysing a specific policy I try to search out its uncertain objectives systematically. Given my doubts about the stability of purposes, I assume that objectives in any public policy are multiple, ambiguous and conflicting.'

Third, in many services clearly valid output measures are not available even were there to be agreement on what desirable outputs might be. The output measures that are being used must therefore first be an object of investigation in their own right. An evaluative design cannot presume that they will be self-evident. Finally, the rational model is misleading in the sharp distinction it draws between means and ends, a distinction which only leads to confusion as evaluators seek to incorporate it in their research designs. Rein (1976, p. 21) stresses the importance of a more flexible approach:

> The relationship between the means and ends of social policy is not settled, nor is it ever likely to be finally resolved. The unsettled nature of social policy, and as a result the study of the interplay between social purposes and how they work out in practice must also be central to the analyst's concern.

Certainly throughout the following chapters of this book we shall be demonstrating how aims, assessed needs, inputs, outputs, achievements and feedbacks are by no means either as separate or sequentially related as, for example, Goldberg and Connelly (1982), whom we quoted earlier, seem to suggest.

The presumption of the experimentalist ideal

The second presumption that is frequently made within evaluative research is that of the desirability of experimental or quasi-experimental designs. Cochrane (1972) has been a vocal exponent of the general strengths of this type of study. In the field of the elderly, Goldberg is a major advocate of the merits of this genre, particularly in the light of her own important example of a piece of evaluative research following quasi-experimental designs (Goldberg et al. 1970; Goldberg and Connelly 1982).

The central features of the experiment in the context of evaluating health services have been set out by Illsley (1980). The main objectives of the programme being studied are clarified (or deemed to be clear). The experiment (or randomized controlled trial) tests the intervention against alternatives (including non-action). There are precise measures of, and controls over, the inputs to the programme. The criterion of success is unidimensional and uncontroversial. Extraneous variables can be excluded or controlled.

In spite of the obvious advantages of the approach, both Goldberg and Illsley have pointed to considerable difficulties. Random assignment of clients to different services is seldom possible. There are ethical as well as administrative objections to randomization. Practitioners learn as they go along so that inputs to the programmes are rarely stable through the experiment. Professionals operating the service also become aware of the different treatments and this introduces a bias. Even at their most successful such research projects compare only two programmes rather than the broad range of alternatives, as really required. It is almost impossible in many settings to exclude extraneous variables. (Services are reorganized, there are demographic changes, new institutions are opened, professionals working in the services change, and so on.) Usually measures of success are equivocal. Even supposing that the problems that we have just mentioned are overcome, the experiment or controlled trial can say very little about *why* any changes that may have been detected have occurred.

Rein (1983) lists one further and especially significant difficulty: that of establishing the character of the service that is being studied within the experiment. Following Hyman and Wright (1968), Rein notes (p. 162):

> An important aspect of an evaluation, then, is examination of what the program is. Finding out a program's intent begins with the program's rhetoric. Getting beneath the rhetoric to the realities of intent and interest is another question. Defining a program is difficult when there is little agreement on the activities to be included or on the intent that unifies those activities into a coherent purpose. Since the 'activity' to be evaluated is not self-evident, it must be treated as problematic, rather than established.

So there is a considerable degree of agreement on the difficulties of the experimental approach. However, although there is this agreement, quite different conclusions are drawn. Goldberg and Connelly, for example, regard 'the randomized experiment or at least an approximation of it' as a 'most powerful tool' and insist that difficulties are surmountable and the potential rewards considerable. They suggest that the relatively few quasi-experimental studies that have been conducted are of great interest because they come closer than other designs to assessing the actual effects of specific types of social care. They admit that 'the harvest is yet small' but insist that this should be no discouragement since 'these studies have prepared some of the appropriate methods and tools for doing the job' (Goldberg and Connelly 1982, p. 248). Although they concede that some objections to the experimental ideal are difficult to meet, they insist that many 'can be overcome by careful preparatory work *with the practitioners who are going to participate in the experiment*'.

Illsley, on the other hand, argues that even if some of the practical difficulties are 'in theory, superable by refinements of technique, design or negotiation' *in practice* that is rarely so. He points out that typically four sets of circumstances inhibit the use of rigorous experimental evaluation. These are (1980 p. 115):

1. Inability to determine goals
2. Inability to control output
3. Inability to measure or evaluate output
4. A combination of 1, 2 and 3.

Illsley is also more cautious about the potential for solving problems in conjunction with service practitioners. He notes that many failures in evaluative work are attributable to the different perspectives of service providers and scientific research workers. In order to satisfy the requirements of the experimental design, research workers frequently impose conditions upon the routine provision of service which create administrative, ethical and clinical complications. These produce resistance to evaluation, and tension between evaluator and service-provider: 'Regrettably the interests of the two do not always coincide.' (Illsley 1980, pp. 115–116). It is not that Illsley does not value practitioner-researcher collaboration. Quite the contrary. He insists that evaluation and the feedback of results should be a central part of service provision. But the social world of health and welfare services is simply not the controlled setting of the experimental laboratory or the trial of a new drug. Indeed, as Cronbach et al. (1980, p. 318) point out, the attempt by evaluators to conform to what many planners and professionals see as the experimental ideal, is counter-productive and serves only to sour relationships.

> Disillusion is the bitter aftertaste of saccharine illusion. It is self-defeating to aspire to deliver an evaluative conclusion as precise and as safely beyond dispute as an operational-language conclusion from the laboratory. It is unrealistic to hope to tell the PSC [policy-shaping community] all it needs to know. When the evaluator aspires only to provide clarification that would not otherwise be available, he has chosen a task he can manage and one that does have social benefits.

The presumption of consensus

The third presumption that is frequently made within evaluative research is that which we may term the presumption of consensus in professional organization. Pervading the whole approach of traditional evaluation is an imagery of unity. We have already referred to the way in which an organizational goal and a clear statement of 'the' policy is central to many evaluative designs. As Silverman (1979, p. 9) points out in his criticism of traditional modes of organizational analysis: 'It seems doubtful whether it is legitimate to conceive of an organization as having a goal except where there is an ongoing consensus between the members of the organization about the purposes of their interaction.'

But the presumption of consensus in evaluative research goes further than this. It extends to the insistence that some agreed criteria of success must serve as the basis for the evaluation, that there is some 'right' or 'objective' view of what is happening within the programme, and that it is the task of the evaluator to establish this objectivity. And, as House (1980, pp. 54–55) points out, intersubjective *agreement* between the parties to the programme is frequently taken as the exclusive indicator of this objectivity. Thus,

> There is a sense in which the intersubjective verification principle is carried through to the definition of goals as well as in the measurement of efforts. It is assumed in the managerial approach to valuation that one can reach a consensus on the goals of a particular project. This assumption is critical .... for the consensus defines what the evaluation will look for.

This consensus frequently does not exist. Yet because evaluators presume that it does they commit the error, which has been so prevalent in organization analysis (Allbrow 1968), of equating the interest of the institution as a whole with the interests of senior managers and officials. Cronbach et al. (1980, p. 84) explain:

> The theory of evaluation ... has been developed almost wholly around the image of command. It is supposed that information flows to a manager or policy official who has a firm grasp on the controls. She can reach a 'correct' decision and act on it. Actually, however, most action is determined by a pluralistic community, not by a lone decision maker. Parties having divergent perceptions and aims bear down on law makers and administrators ... When there are multiple participants with multiple views, it is meaningless to speak of one action as the rational or correct action. The active parties jockey towards a politically acceptable accommodation.

This line of argument suggests the need to develop a more pluralistic approach which could cope with diversity and conflict. A more subjectivist methodology would promote the collection of multiple perspectives on the programme (not necessarily in agreement with each other) and would incorporate them into the evaluation exercise. Ambiguity and lack of agreement in perception between

parties of the policy-shaping community would then be a central feature of the research, rather than an embarrassment as is the case when the presumption of consensus prevails.

These, then, are three important presumptions contained within much evaluative research. Our view is that a methodology based upon them has generated problems. It has made evaluators irritated at the apparent reluctance of their research subjects to behave rationally, define their goals clearly, and the like. Sometimes researchers have taken on these tasks themselves and there are examples of whole programmes of research which, in consequence, have become bogged down in trying to define and clarify the object of their study (BIOSS 1974; Billis et al. 1980). Evaluators have also been confused as they sought to cope with a plurality of perspectives on the meanings of 'success' and they became frustrated as they found themselves unable to effect the controls of the experimental setting.

New directions

We are by no means the first to note the difficulties that we have described or to make criticisms of what has been the predominant approach to evaluative research. A number of suggestions have been made about the new directions which evaluative methodology should now take.

Studying process

In response to the comment that many evaluations do not explain *why* a particular outcome occurs, Robertson and Gandy (1983, pp. 246 and 249), amongst others, have drawn the distinction between outcome evaluation and process evaluation:

> Outcome evaluations attempt to assess the effects produced by policies or programmes, and the extent to which such results measure up to programme 'goals' (however these may be defined). As such, they perhaps come closest to the scientific ideal of verification – and it is probably this fact which best explains their still burgeoning popularity. . . . From a methodological point of view, process evaluations are rather less glamorous exercises than evaluations of outcome; and it is possibly for this reason that few investigations of this type seem to be undertaken or reported in the literature. The purpose of process research is to identify – normally through the use of 'soft' methodologies like participant observation – what seem to be the most important elements contributory to the outcomes of any given programme, and the way these elements relate to each other within the policy or treatment-programme itself . . . This kind of research is therefore reliant on description and inference from observation, in order to build up a sensitive composite picture of the functioning of a programme.

Illuminative evaluation

House (1980, p. 41), quoting Parlett and Hamilton's research in the field of education, describes what he calls 'illuminative evaluation':

> The aim of illuminative evaluation is to study the program; how it operates, how it is influenced by the situation in which it is applied; what those directly concerned regard as its advantages and disadvantages; and how students' intellectual tasks

> and academic experiences are most affected. 'It aims to discover and document what it is like to be participating in the scheme, whether as a teacher or pupil, and, in addition, to discern and discuss the innovation's most significant features, returning concomitants and critical processes. (Parlett and Hamilton, 1977: 19)

Illsley (1980) describes a study by Hunter (1980) as an example of 'illuminative evaluation'. The Hunter study examined the impact of central government policy on imbalances between health authorities and between care groups and sectors of care within authorities. Hunter focussed on the process by which financial resources were allocated to different ends and Illsley highlights several features of this study. The data 'differed considerably from the conventional data of scientific trials' and were derived from notes on observed meetings, structured interviews, and 'casual chat around corridors and canteens' as well as from questionnaires and committee documents. The research pursued several loose hypotheses and was multiparadigmatic in approach. The project also studied the process of decision making, as it occurred, over time. Thus, 'The data are not cut and dried in the tradition of the natural sciences, instead they trace and reflect what is and must be a fragmented, complex process.'

In terms of the traditional approach to evaluation, research such as this could not be described as evaluative study. It is nevertheless of considerable help in answering crucial evaluative questions about the allocation of resources. Illsley (p. 135) concludes:

> I consider that, as scientific attention turns from laboratory conditions and drug or operative intervention to the study of health services and policy change, where formal trials are most often impracticable or unrevealing, sociological research of this kind will become increasingly for evaluative purposes necessary. [*sic*]

Subjectivist epistemology

Growing interest in subjectivist and phenomenological approaches within the social sciences (e.g. following Berger and Luckman 1967) has also begun to influence suggestions about new directions for evaluative research. Studies in a number of different fields of service provision, based upon a broadly similar theoretical framework, have examined what have been referred to as 'ideologies' (Hardiker 1977; Smith 1980), 'models' (May 1971), 'assumptive worlds' (Young and Mills 1978) and 'frames of relevance' (Asquith 1977) to depict the perspective of professionals and officials responsible for policy formation and implementation. House (1980, p. 57) comments and explains the pertinence of these approaches to evaluative research:

> The subjectivists are less interested in arriving at a proposition that is 'true' (in the generalizable sense) than in relating the evaluation to the particular experience of the audience. They attempt to obtain valid insights within the frame of reference of the group for whom they are working. It is assumed that there is a gap between language and experience. Tacit rather than explicit knowledge is what the evaluator seeks. The evaluation is intentionally context-bound, and findings are interpreted in context. Since the audience may well have a firmer grasp of the context, based on greater experience, the audience's interpretation of an event may be superior to that of an evaluator. Subjectivist evaluators are more concerned in their work with

> specific causal statements (internal validity) than with general causal statements (external validity).

Methodologically such an approach has several implications. Data collection tends to be naturalistic. There is a preference for loosely structured interviews, observations and field notes based on informal participation. Both collection and analysis of data attempt to explore the interrelationship between subjective perspectives and operational policies, and throughout data collection, attention to a variety of perspectives is crucial. This dictates attention to a variety of data sources. House (1980, p. 57) summarizes:

> The evaluator tries to collect multiple perspectives, although the perspectives may not agree with each other. Historical investigation and the following of events over time are also critical. The historical mode of investigation is more appropriate than the natural science mode. Emphasis is on the qualitative rather than the quantitative.

This allusion to a pluralistic stance is one that warrants listing below in its own right.

Political and methodological pluralism

So far in this chapter we have on several occasions noted the importance of a pluralistic approach both in the attention to be paid to varied data sources and in the weight to be assigned to the varied perceptions and interests of the numerous groups which are party to the policy process. House (1980, p. 127) makes the link between pluralism, evaluation, and a number of themes which have arisen in our discussion so far:

> [Pluralists] value the participation of the people involved in the program. Generally, this participation consists of collecting the viewpoints and opinions of various people about the program or policy issue. The evaluator faithfully records and portrays their viewpoints. In this manner, the principles, criteria, and weightings of the people involved are used to judge the program ...
>
> In portraying the judgements of various groups associated with the program, this latter approach is pluralist not only in the philosophical sense of judging on the basis of several principles but also pluralist in the political sense of representing different political interests.

This perspective will be particularly, although by no means exclusively, influential through the rest of this book and we shall be returning to it in general terms in the final chapter. At this stage in the discussion, however, Cronbach et al. (1980) provides just one illustration of the impact of pluralistic perspectives on evaluative research. They set out ninety-five theses geared to the reform of programme evaluation and directly influenced by the 'political theory of "pluralistic social research"'. The following are several of these theses:

> 11. A theory of evaluation must be as much a theory of political interaction as it is a theory of how to determine facts. ...
> 23. An image of pluralistic accommodation more truly represents how policy and programs are shaped than does the Platonic image of concentrated power and responsibility. ...
> 38. Strictly honest data collection can generate a misleading picture unless ques-

> tions are framed to expose both the facts useful to partisans of the program and the facts useful to its critics. . . .
> 54. It is better for an evaluative inquiry to launch a small fleet of studies than to put all its resources into a single approach. . . .
> 64. Multiple indicators of outcomes reinforce one another logically as well as statistically. This is true for measures of adequacy of program implementations as well as for measures of changes in client behaviour.

Taken together these suggestions that we have reviewed in this section mark, tentatively, some new directions for evaluative research. The notion that there is a neat stereotype for an evaluation design is discredited. Research which has not previously been regarded as conforming to an evaluative format may nevertheless contain the data that are required to answer evaluative questions. Evaluative research must pay much more attention to evaluating the ways in which policy is formulated and implemented. An understanding of these processes is part and parcel of policy evaluation. The policy as subjectively perceived by the participants to the policy process is also critical. Moreover the plurality of perspectives and operating tactics at work within these processes calls for attention to detail and the collection of varied data sources as a key feature of the methodology of evaluative research.

Conclusion

In opening this chapter we suggested that several problems have arisen in evaluating social care because of the presumptions that have been made about the rational character of the policy process within health and welfare agencies, because of the commitment which many studies have shown to an experimental approach, and because the presumption of consensus in professional organizations has diverted attention away from the plurality of perspectives which participants hold on service provision. In conclusion we shall outline the broad features of an approach to studying new provisions which, we suggest, may avoid some of these difficulties and which takes seriously the way in which *multiple* criteria of success features in the innovation of services.

We shall be drawing upon several strands of the various suggestions that have been made for a 'new approach' to evaluative research. We have termed our approach 'pluralistic evaluation'. The central point we are making is that if we are to understand and evaluate the part played by the several different groups involved in the care of a client group then we must understand how they use different criteria of success in their own interests and how 'success' thus operates in the social context of its use. Evaluative research must therefore not only evaluate 'success' but also *explore and explain* the institution (be it hospital, social work agency, or whatever) and its services. The approach is heavily informed by models of institutional functioning and the policy process which draw upon theories of political pluralism (Hall et al. 1975; cf. also McGrew et al., eds. 1982, Weale, 1983). We also find an 'incrementalist' picture (Lindblom 1959) of the policy process to be a more convincing account than the rational models which pervade management thought. Our approach is influenced too by that 'subjectivist' tradition of research within sociology which takes the actors' 'definition of the situation' as a starting-point for investigation.

It follows from these standpoints that, first, evaluative research must identify the major constituent groups to the policy initiative with which it is concerned and, throughout the research, compare these groups with each other, both in their ideological perspectives and in their operational strategies. Secondly, the approach directs us to collect data on these groups' interpretations and perceptions of 'success' in service provision and assign to that data a central place in the evaluative analysis. Thirdly, the study must document not only the plurality of notions of 'success' but also the different groups' strategies as they strive to implement their own perspectives in their own interests. Fourthly, evaluative research must then assess the extent to which success (or failure) is achieved on each of the several criteria employed and in terms of the several meanings assigned to these criteria. Success is a pluralistic notion. It is not a unitary measure. In consequence, fifthly, pluralistic evaluation must embody the principles of methodological triangulation. Denzin (1978a) has argued that any study dependent upon a single data source is 'method bound'. The point of particular relevance to evaluation research is that each data source is interest bound (as tied to the perspective of one group rather than that of another). The constant use of as great a variety of different kinds of data as possible ensures, so far as possible, that the research reflects the full range of interests, ideologies, interpretations and achievements abroad within the agency. Thus, sixthly, pluralistic evaluation generates both an ethnography of the way in which the services develop and an explanation of this development (in terms of the pluralistic interest of participating groups). It is central to policy evaluation to attempt to link the problems of an organization as perceived by its constituents, to the performance of the institution's programme of service.

Evaluative research embodying these points certainly seems to have some important advantages. It is likely to show that in some ways a service is successful and in some ways it is not. That may seem trite. However, it is an advance on the substantial body of organizational research which shows that most organizations simply fail to live up to their utopian ideals. We need to be more precise than that. There is also the point that an inability to show *why* particular failures or successes occur is a frequent weakness in evaluative research. Pluralistic evaluation says a good deal about why some outcomes but not others take place. This opens the way to proposals for change. There is little point in knowing that a service ranks high or low on some criterion, however supposedly 'objective', if we cannot conclude from the analysis how the performance can be improved. It is important to remember that even high levels of success may have significant costs in terms of unanticipated consequences. Many evaluative strategies have no way of detecting these costs. Although the strategy that we have suggested is by no means perfect on this count, its more diverse approach means that it stands greater chance of revealing the unplanned as well as the planned outcomes of innovation in providing services.

There is also the question of implementation. Any recommendations for improvement will depend for implementation, at least in part, upon the attitude of agency members to the evaluation exercise. Many evaluations are dismissed because they do not use the criteria which the several groups in the agency themselves employ. While pluralistic evaluation may seem complex and uncertain in its use of multiple criteria, it cannot be dismissed for failure to take at least some account of the perspective of any significant group of participants. While most 'objective' evaluation seeks to remain politically neutral but in practice becomes hopelessly embroiled in the politics of the organization being studied (even if the evaluators do not always realize what is happening), pluralistic evaluation stands some chance of remaining 'independent' and 'neutral' by having taken sympathetic account of as many perspectives as possible. By taking the political processes of the agency seriously there is some chance that the political role of evaluation itself will be clarified. As we have argued throughout this introductory chapter, little is to be gained by pretending that the dynamics of pursuing and evaluating success are simpler than they really are.

CHAPTER TWO

A New Psychogeriatric Day Hospital

Introduction

In this chapter we describe the setting for our research, outlining the main features of a day hospital which is the object of the evaluation. The chapter presents background material for the rest of the book. Through this description of the hospital we shall also highlight in specific terms the difficulties of designing evaluative research which we discussed more generally in Chapter 1.

Development of the hospital

The day hospital which is the subject of our study is (according to information produced by the health authority for patients' relatives and for related professions) intended to help maintain and increase the level of independence of elderly persons with mental disorder and to provide help and support for patients in the community, for their families and for health and related professions who provide community services.

It was a very important aspect of the launching of this institution that a considerable air of innovation pervaded the whole planning process. The area in which the hospital is sited is not one which has been known in the past for very progressive health care in the psychiatric field and planners made frequent reference to the day hospital not only as a new institution but also as a new institution of a new kind; something which was unusual in the area. From an early stage there was widespread support for the view that the hospital should be evaluated. Thus in many respects an account of the early history of the hospital is an account of the early history of the research project also (cf. Werry et al. 1974).

The criteria to be used in this evaluation, however, were not clear. The working party planning the hospital noted (somewhat categorically) that, 'Members of the working party did not have a shared idea of the objectives of the day hospital.' It was suggested only that 'evaluaters ought to determine the effectiveness of provision measured against relevant criteria', although an impression of the range of criteria considered to be relevant at that early stage can be gained from some of the items which were on the agenda for evaluation: liaison with GPs, criteria for admission and discharge, links with related community services, staff morale, family involvement, transportation and cost. It was also noted that a later meeting would 'arrive at a shared view of the objectives of the day hospital'. As we shall be describing, negotiating consensus is a more complex process than that.

Initial plans

The original impetus for building this hospital came from the area executive group, working within overall health board policy, and under considerable pressure from both consultant psychiatrists and senior administrators to increase the provision in the region for elderly patients with mental disorder. The working party mentioned above was established to examine urgently the feasibility of establishing, in the short term, day hospital facilities for this category of patients. It produced a first report in 1978.

From the start of these deliberations it was clear that existing provision was inadequate. Projections based upon the 1976 Registrar-General's data indicated that, although over the following ten years there would be a 4.5% increase of only approximately 48,500 to 50,000 persons over 65 in the health board area and of only about 26,600 to 28,000 (around 4.7%) in the relevant district, the district population over 75 would rise from 9,000 to about 13,500 (about 49%). The working party reported the common observation that 'the risk of psychiatric disorder manifesting itself in the latter grouping is disproportionately high and, due to their relative longevity, the majority of patients are female.' On the basis of these figures it was argued that 120 day-hospital places were needed and then only (a) to cope with the current and not projected population and (b) to serve as 'a palliative measure to cope with chronic bed shortages which would support patients and their families where no other suitable means were available'. (This kind of conclusion, based on these kinds of data, is very usual: see Carver and Liddiard 1978, part 1; Kinnaird et al. 1981, section 1.) The working party made the point that the use of a day hospital as an *alternative* to in-patient beds departed from the usual practice of treating day hospitals as a *complement* to in-patient and community health facilities.

On the basis of existing waiting-list data, a case was made for a 40-place day hospital as an interim measure, pending the establishment of a 120-bed hospital with a purpose-built day hospital attached as an additional facility. It was anticipated that patients using the new day hospital would be mainly 'patients with chronic brain syndromes, i.e. dementias' and 'patients with functional (non-organic) psychiatric illnesses, i.e. depressives, schizophrenics, neuroses of old age', divided female to male in approximately the ratio 5:1. Given the level and type of demand, a significant number of places was necessary to make the venture worthwhile and 'the regime must be geared to rehabilitation, otherwise the number of patients able to benefit will be restricted by a conspicuous lack of throughput'.

Several sites were investigated as possible locations for a new unit. Amongst the factors influencing the choice were, of course, time and cost, but also accessibility of existing services, existing staff attitudes and orientations, longer-term plans for a 120-bed in-patient unit, the likely ability of the new hospital to provide a rehabilitative service to in-patients and the problems of providing transport. Problems with transport arose because the ambulance service required eighteen months' notice for new demands of this kind – and anyway preliminary investigation, combined with the lessons learned from visiting some other day hospitals, indicated that ambulance provision was far from ideal. Under such arrangements patients tended to arrive late and leave early and transport was subject to disruption if more urgent calls upon the ambulances arose. To overcome these difficulties the health board agreed initially to bear the costs of transport and several possible arrangements were investigated, including the use of a health board mini-bus and the use of commercial coach companies. In the event a contract was awarded to a local coach operator and the cost of this contract was later transferred to the ambulance services.

The outcome of the working party's deliberations was a proposal for a prefabricated structure on the site of an older hospital (Park Hospital), designed to last as a day hospital for perhaps as little as five years (although with a life as a building of some twenty years) depending upon plans for a new unit and the future of the older hospital itself (cf. Cosin 1971).

Overall then, the day hospital was planned as a modern and innovative programme and staff and health board officials pointed from the start to features of the institution which were regarded as placing it in the forefront of psychogeriatric care. The hospital was designed to avoid 'silt up' (where few new vacances ever occur) of its patient population. Stress was placed on the importance of individual assessment and treatment for each patient. Social work services were intended to play a distinctive and active role in the hospital. Transport arrangements were unusually good. The hospital was planned to bring together an especially wide range of different services (cf. Berger and Berger 1971).

By May 1979 building work was in progress with the target, which was met, of the hospital becoming operational in October of that year. The total capital cost of the scheme was approximately £79,000. The revenue consequences were to amount to some £65,700 (at 1979 prices) inclusive of staffing, supplies and services, and patient transport. The new day hospital was officially opened in November 1979.

Continuing developments

As the places in the hospital began to fill up during the first few months of its operation and as it began to discharge patients as well as admit them, it became, like all innovating institutions, an organization continually changing in numerous ways. Our research covered in all a period of some three years and in later chapters we refer to some changes which took place during this time.

However even after this period of consolidation (and after most of our data were collected) changes continued to occur. For example, a new general district hospital was opened in the area with additional facilities for geriatric patients. New job oportunities created by this new hospital also led to considerable staff movement within the area. The local social work department ceased using 'Part 4' accommodation (for elderly clients in its care) in Park Hospital and the reorganization of work occasioned by this development was taken as an opportunity to rearrange nursing officer and ward sister responsibilities. Two new community nurses were also appointed to visit discharged or non-attending patients of the day hospital.

Perhaps most important of all, a reorganization of the psychiatric services in the area (described as 'sectorization') gave responsibility for all psychogeriatric cases in a district around the day hospital to one consultant psychogeriatrician. A joint waiting list was established for beds in Park Hospital and a nearby psychiatric hospital. This made the transfer of patients between beds in different hospitals and between the day hospital and other hospitals somewhat easier.

These and other changes mean that had we collected our data at a different time some of our specific observations would have been different. Since all organizations (especially innovations) change, that it always true of institutional research. However, we do not believe that our general conclusions would have differed significantly because our methods of data collection and our theoretical approach to evaluation are not based upon the assumption of a static object of analysis. We have attempted to take into account a continual process of change as an intrinsic part of our research approach.

The day hospital

The building

The hospital is a modern, purpose-built construction opened by one of the Scottish health authorities in the autumn of 1979 and situated in the grounds of a larger and much older hospital (Park Hospital) which caters for geriatric, psychogeriatric and a range of adult mentally subnormal in-patients, many of whom are long-term residents. The buildings of Park Hospital originally accommodated the work house for the area and still hold something of the 'poor's-house' imagery in the town. Figure 1 is a sketch map showing the location of the day hospital on the Park Hospital site.

Internally the large 'activity area' of the day hospital is carpeted (unusual in hospitals where not all patients are continent) and comfortably furnished. Smaller rooms include a kitchen, cloakrooms, treatment room, bedroom and bath and shower rooms (cf. Ellis 1974). Visitors are almost always impressed with the appearance of the hospital. Figure 2 is a sketch plan of the layout of the hospital's main facilities.

The hospital site is on the outskirts of the town and, since patients attending the hospital are drawn from a dispersed and largely rural geographical area, patient transport is crucial. Each morning and evening a coach makes two circular tours to collect and then return home those patients who are attending

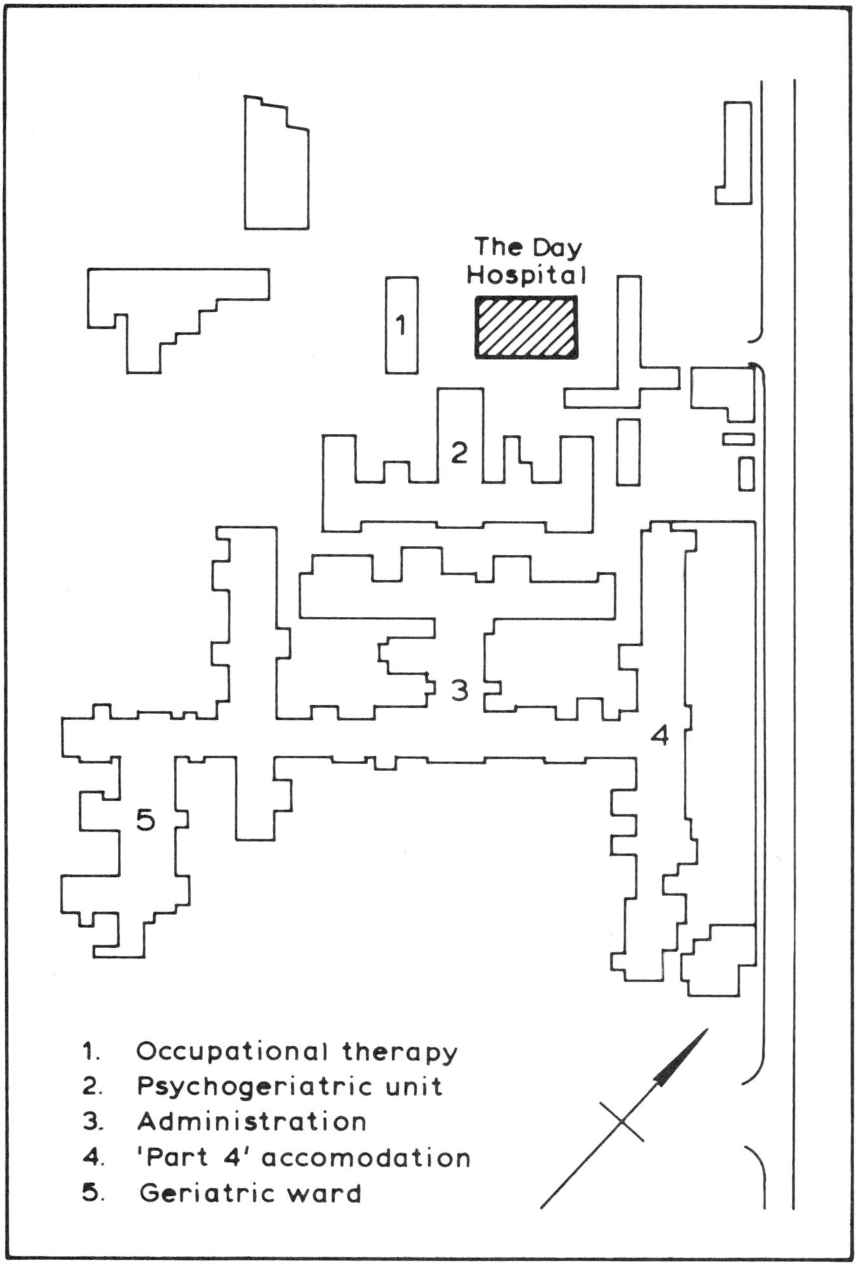

Figure 1 The day hospital on the Park Hospital site

Figure 2 The day hospital: accommodation

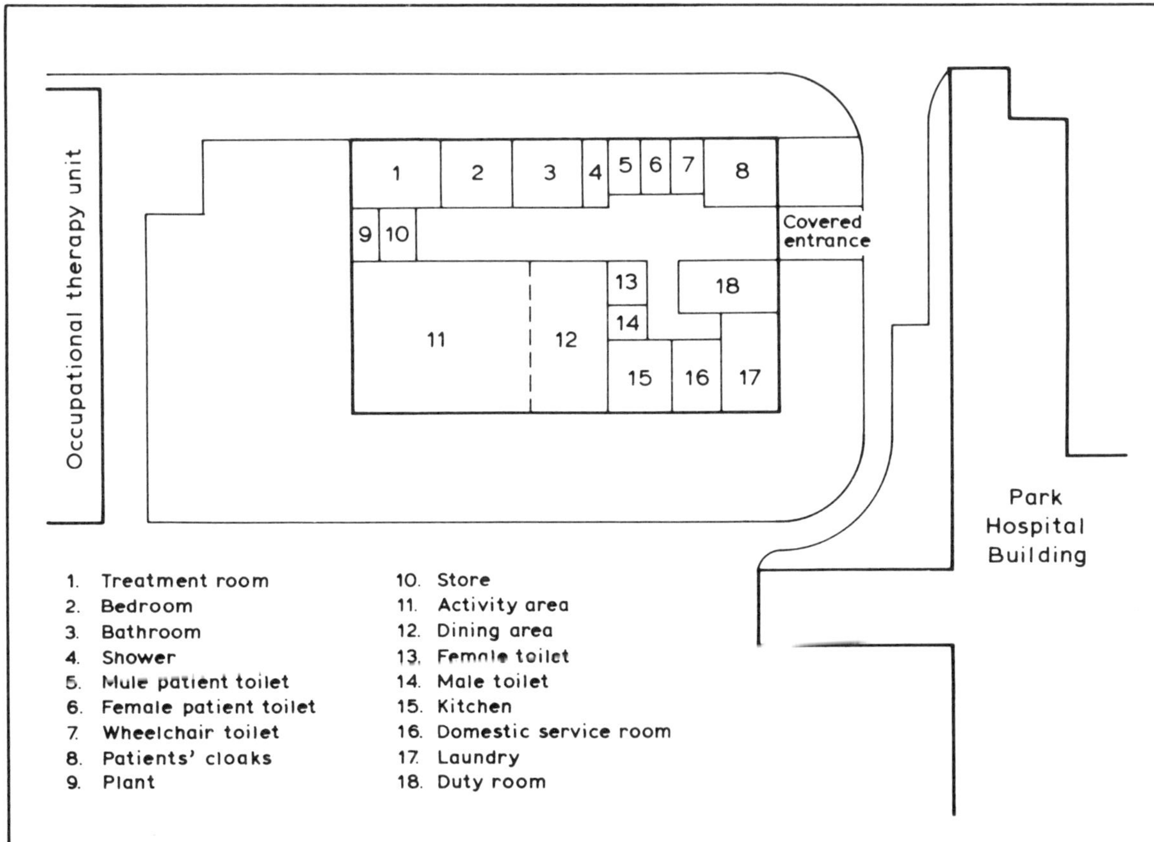

but who do not have their own transport. This ensures that no patient spends less than six hours at the hospital on each of their days of attendance.

One novel feature of the scheme is that nursing auxiliaries accompany the coach driver (cf. Hildick-Smith 1974). They attend to patients during the journey and also accompany them between the coach and their homes. Thus the nurses can check, for example, that lighting and heating have been correctly turned off before the patient leaves the house. The idea is that the journey itself becomes a part of the 'treatment'. Hospital staff learn more of the patient's home background, and patients living alone who might otherwise need relatives to 'see them off' in the morning, can, in this way, attend the hospital without the attentions of an 'informal carer'.

Patients

Approximately twenty-five patients each day attend the hospital. It is open weekdays only. Patients attend for between one and five days each week and in any one week some thirty-five patients attend.

There is considerable variation amongst patients in the type and extent of family support which is available to them at home but relatives do play a significant part in the care of about 75% of all patients. About 30% of all patients actually live with a spouse and around 25% of all patients live with other relatives. Greene and Timbury (1979) have a similar finding. Barber and Wallis (1976) report that 50% of 'caring relatives' live with the patient (see also Carver and Liddiard (eds. 1978, part 3)).

An interim report of the working party on the development of the hospital stated:

> Patients could fall within any of the categories:
> 2.4.1 Patients with chronic brain syndrome, i.e. dementias.
> 2.4.2 Patients with functional (non-organic) illness, i.e. depressions, schizophrenics, neuroses of old age.
> 2.4.3 Patients with acute brain syndromes, mainly toxic confusional states or deliria.
> 2.4.4 Patients with long-standing psychiatric illnesses usually found as a 'graduate' group in mental hospitals.
> It has been assumed that the majority of patients will fall particularly into category 2.4.1 and to some extent into 2.4.2 but we feel that a day hospital should be available to care for all types of elderly patients with mental disability, provided they are ambulant.

The major criteria that are advanced by consultants and other staff for admitting patients to the day hospital are that those admitted will be over sixty-four years old and have had a history of psychiatric illness. The way in which specific patients are selected for hospital attendance is as follows.

In general patients must be referred to the consultant-in-charge from the patient's GP. The initial impetus may come from the GP himself/herself or from the patient (rarely), relatives (more often) or staff of sheltered housing, residential accommodation or some other service. As well as referrals which specifically mention the desirability of day hospital attendance some referrals from GPs request a more general psychiatric assessment of the patient or consideration for short- or long-term admission to an in-patient bed. The consultant may also consider some patients from the current in-patient population of related hospitals for a day hospital place. (As we shall see in Chapter 3, this point is important methodologically since the practice of this day hospital means that not all cases considered for admission are 'referrals' in the usual sense of that term.)

The decision on admission is made by the consultant psychiatrist, frequently with the benefit of a domiciliary visit, often with the added benefit of a report on a domiciliary visit from the social worker attached to the day hospital and usually in consultation with other staff at a weekly meeting. Some referrals require no decision because they 'drop out' through changes in their circumstances or because patients or relatives refuse to consider attendance. The decision to admit is a complex one that we shall be discussing in greater detail in later chapters. It is certainly not just a function of the patients' age and diagnosed psychiatric disorder.

In the early stages of the hospital's operation about 65% of the patients admitted suffered, in varying degrees, from organic dementia although the proportion of such cases and their severity tended to increase over the period of the research. Patients with depressive illnesses account for about 20% of admissions and patients with schizophrenic, paranoid or essentially physical disorders are represented in small numbers. The problems which patients present are described in records as including aggression, wandering, incontinence, inability to cope with the electricity, gas or fires, mood disturbance, hallucinations, general forgetfulness and inability to communicate.

Patients must be physically fit enough to be able to attend and may not be admitted if, for example, they are aggressive towards other patients (although Watts and Bennett (1978) argue that violence and poor social integration show no relation to outcome.)

As with the admission decision, the decision to discharge a patient also involves a range of organizational and other variables which we later document.

Figures 3–5 present a picture of the flow of patients through the hospital. The data are taken from our 14-month sample which is discussed fully in Chapter 3. Figure 3 is a flow chart indicating relative numbers of patients following different career paths through the hospital. Figure 4 gives the duration of attendance of patients discharged during the sample period. Figure 5 gives the duration of attendance of the patient population at the end of this period.

We shall be discussing patient flow in greater detail in a subsequent chapter but, in our 'working description' of the hospital, the following broad conclusions seemed tenable. First, there is considerable movement of patients into and out of the hospital and little evidence of the service 'silting up'. Second, although a range of different disposals are in operation, a rather high proportion of patients enter long-term care after day hospital attendance. Third, although the day hospital has interchange arrangements with a number of other institutions, by far and away the most significant amount of interchange is with short-term beds

Figure 3 The day hospital: patient flow during initial fourteen-month period

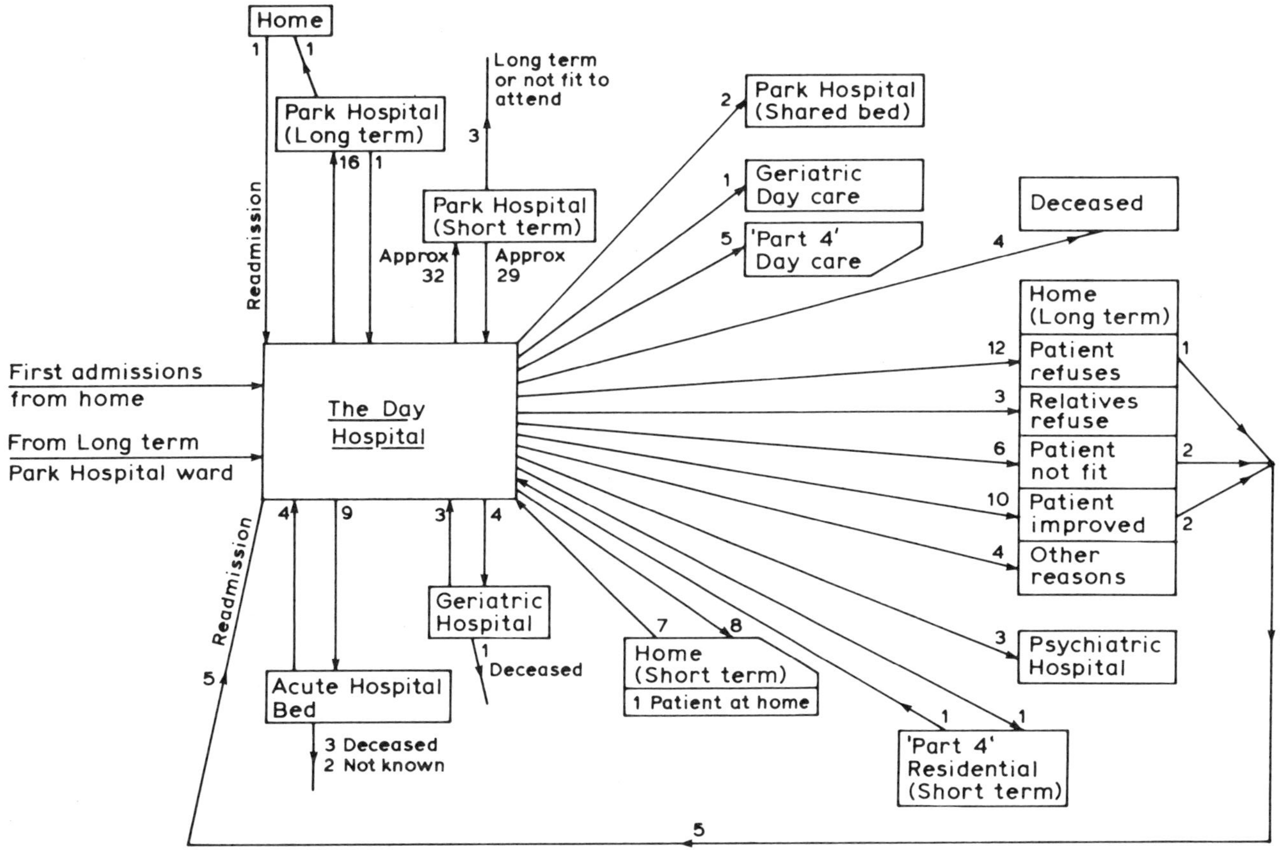

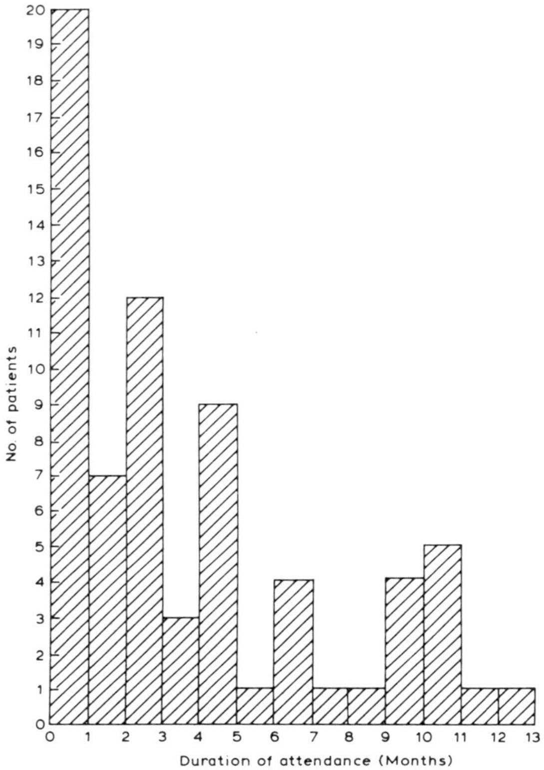

Figure 4 The day hospital: duration of first attendance in initial fourteen-month period

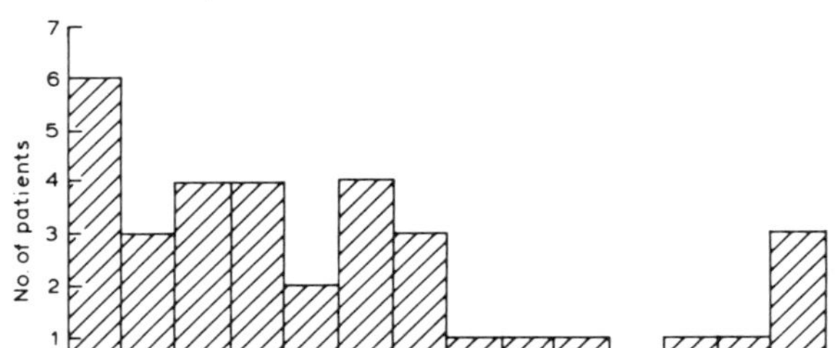

Figure 5 The day hospital: duration of attendance at the end of initial fourteen-month period

in Park Hospital. Fourth, the day hospital does not function to any great extent as a stepping stone for patients leaving long-term hospital accommodation and returning home. Fifth, although a majority of discharged patients have attended the hospital for less than three months, amongst the population of the hospital at any one time a clear *minority* will be short-stay patients. If patients are divided by diagnosis into dementia and non-dementia categories, then at any one time dementia patients account for some 50% of cases since, although a large number of the 65% of admissions which are diagnosed dementias are discharged fairly quickly, amongst those who remain for a lengthy period dementias are highly represented.

Staffing

The staff which, it was considered, would be necessary to operate the new hospital, and the duties that they would perform were described in considerable detail in a set of 'operational policies' drawn up by health board administrators in consultation with their professional advisers.

The core care staff consists of consultant psychiatrist, medical officer, sister (charge nurse), senior enrolled nurse, social worker and community nurse (cf. Peace 1980). The consultant, based at another psychiatric hospital, is responsible for providing psychiatric care to patients, for decisions regarding acceptance and discharge, for leading the multiprofessional team, and for keeping under continuous review the work of the hospital in relation to the needs of the health board for psychogeriatric services. The consultant is assisted by a GP working at the day hospital as medical officer on a sessional basis. Within the overall charge of a senior nursing officer at Park Hospital, the sister and senior enrolled nurse are in charge of the day-to-day nursing administration of the unit. They are assisted by two part-time enrolled nurses (1.25 whole-time equivalents) and five nursing assistants (three whole-time equivalents - generally referred to as the 'nursing auxiliaries'). The social worker, formally accountable to a senior social worker in another hospital, is responsible for social background reports on prospective patients, liaison with relatives and links with the social work department and other social work services. The community nurse also makes some home visits. Secretarial and clerical support to nurses and the consultant is provided by a part-time secretary.

Figure 6 is an organization chart of the hospital which gives an overview of links between staff and between the hospital and some related organizations. (Like all charts of this kind it should be read with caution since it is essentially prescriptive and, as we shall show, in practice many of the relationships are more complex than 'lines of accountability' imply).

Figure 6 The day hospital: organization chart

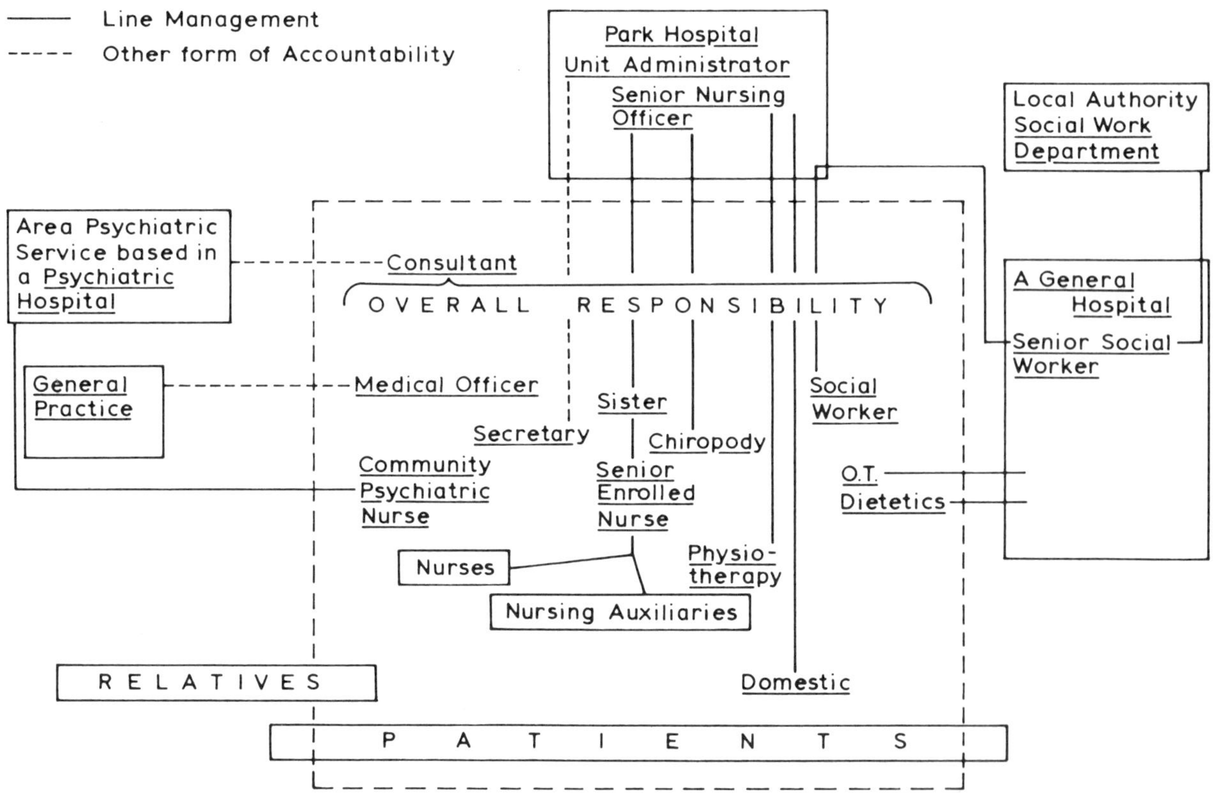

In addition to the services provided by the core staff, professionals, mainly based at Park Hospital, also provide patients with occupational therapy, physiotherapy, chiropody, speech therapy and dental services. For some periods the day hospital has commanded the services of a full-time occupational therapist. There have also been periods when, in practice, it has been difficult to provide some paramedical services, especially dental services.

It is undoubtedly an important feature of the hospital that social work services are more central to its operation than to many other psychogeriatric day hospitals. Although there was initially some expectation that the social worker attached to the day hospital would also provide a social work service to Park Hospital patients, in practice the vast majority of her time is concerned with the day hospital.

Since the social worker is an employee of the local authority's social work department and not of the National Health Service, this position also illustrates the way in which the institution has very 'permeable' boundaries (Smith 1979). Indeed, what counts as the boundary of the day hospital is ambiguous.

Staff meetings

The 'Tuesday meeting', held weekly and attended by senior and some other staff, is partly staff meeting and partly case conference. It is central to decision making in the hospital and we describe it in some detail in later chapters. It takes up the major part of the time that the consultant psychiatrist spends at the day hospital. The sister and social worker play very significant roles in this meeting. The meeting is also a key point of contact in the relationship between the day hospital, Park Hospital and other parts of the psychiatric service. Furthermore, the meeting is important in maintaining the 'morale' of the hospital so that it is in this context that the 'success' of the hospital is displayed and its weaknesses disguised. Generally, control and influence over information and decisions at this meeting are symptomatic of the pattern of events in the hospital as a whole. It is in many ways the 'hub' of the hospital as an organizztion.

Those attending the meeting include the psychiatrist, sister, senior enrolled nurse, social worker, community nurse and secretary, as well as the administrator, occupational therapist, chiropodist and ward sisters from relevant wards in Park Hospital. The meeting lasts for the major part of each Tuesday morning although the occupational therapist, chiropodist and ward sisters do not stay for the whole meeting.

The meeting deals with several different kinds of business and is divided into sections. In one section the consultant discusses cases in Park Hospital with ward sisters. Originally these were intended to be the cases for possible day hospital attendance although in practice not all fall into this category. The progress of patients currently attending the day hospital is reviewed with heavy reliance upon sister consulting the 'Kardex' notes. Admissions and discharges are discussed. The social worker usually contributes actively in this section of the meeting. Finally, the consultant uses the meeting to discuss any 'other problems' that are arising in the running of the hospital. He felt that this was an especially important function during the early phase of the hospital's development. This feeling reflects the importance of understanding the hospital as a developing innovation. The way in which the meeting is designed to incoporate the several groups and interests involved in patient care reinforces the pluralistic character of the day hospital as an organization.

Hospital records

As in most health and welfare institutions, the records system of the day hospital is more complex in practice than at first appears (see Wheeler, ed. 1969). In fact there are several records systems reflecting the contribution of the several different professional groups, especially psychiatric, nursing and social work staff.

A wide variety of documents are used to make and justify decisions about patients. There are GP referral letters, psychiatric reports and reports on domiciliary visits, social workers' social assessment reports, nursing notes on patients recording treatment and progress, a medical history compiled by the medical officer, and a patient index listing details of admissions and discharges. Paramedical staff keep their own records. The secretary also keeps an informal note on the business of the Tuesday meetings.

All these records are kept in several different places. The consultant and social worker retain copies of their reports and the social worker also keeps a copy of reports on patients referred to the day hospital but not admitted. These are required in cases, for example, of rereferral. The psychiatrist also holds, at his office in another hospital, the GP referral letters for day hospital patients.

A file on each current case is housed in a filing cabinet in the day hospital duty room as also is the card index on admissions and discharges. One 'Kardex' file holding the nursing notes and another holding the medication records is housed in the duty room but may be used in the treatment room as well. Also, patients are supposed to bring with them to the day hospital a card recording the medicines that they are being prescribed by their GP. The medical records compiled by the medical officer are kept in two transportable units in the day hospital and these papers are put onto the case files when patients are discharged. Files on past day hospital cases are stored in the general office of Park Hospital and day hospital patients transferred to Park Hospital for short- or long-term care are accompanied by their files.

These details are important in obtaining information about individual cases. A full picture is gained only by consulting psychiatric, social work and Park Hospital case records as well as nursing, medication and medical notes (and even then it is not *complete*). The variety of records and their dispersed locations are also indicative of two important features of the day hospital; the variety of perspectives at work within it and the way in which it is meshed into other parts of the medical, psychiatric and social-work systems of care.

The relatives group

A group for the support of patients' relatives is a comparatively novel feature of the hospital's services (cf. Peace 1980) and a description of the working of this group highlights the very varied bases that exist for evaluating the success of the hospital. In particular the problems with which the hospital is concerned appear very different from relatives', as opposed to the professionals', points of view. We shall be describing the relatives group at considerable length in Chapter 10. During the course of the study it became an important source of data, for its meetings revealed not only different perspectives on the hospital but also the interaction and conflict between these perspectives in patterns of social intercourse. It was also the major example of a development which took place after the study began and which had therefore to be incorporated into the design as the research progressed.

Relations with Park Hospital

The relationship between the day hospital and Park Hospital is ambiguous and yet again stresses the variety of expectations about the day hospital's desirable achievements. The planning papers can be read as implying that the day hospital could as well have been sited anywhere. On the other hand, comments about such matters as favourable staff orientation and attitudes, available facilities and treatment of in-patients at the day hospital might be taken to imply that a 'special relationship' was intended between Park Hospital and the day hospital. In the event the interchange of patients, staff and services between the two institutions proved to be significant in the day hospital's development and in our data collection.

Conclusion

In this chapter we have described some features of the day hospital which is the object of our evaluation, as background to the rest of this report. The description which we have presented here should be read as a 'working description' of the hospital. It was based upon our first impressions and upon the inspection of data that we undertook as the research began. We used it as we decided what further information we needed to collect and how we should collect it. This preliminary account will therefore require elaboration and refinement in the light of the data which we shall present in detail through later chapters of the book. Nevertheless from this description of the hospital and its setting we make some general observations.

(1) The hospital offers such a variety of services and involves so many different groups of professionals, as well as patients and relatives, that its objectives are amenable to a very wide range of interpretations. Therefore no single criterion of evaluation will suffice.

(2) The hospital does have some novel features in the provision of day care for the elderly mentally infirm. The degree of experimentation that is apparent - for example, in opening hours, the relatives group, the role of social work and transport arrangements - adds weight to our view that a major task lies in documenting the nature of the service as a central part of evaluating it. As we have indicated, a pluralistic approach to evaluative research dictates a constant interaction between (a) a description of the innovation, (b) decisions about data collection and research methods, and (c) evaluative conclusions reached through

the analysis of these data. Such an approach contrasts with a more orthodox stance in which an account of the innovation on the one hand and an assessment of the innovation on the other are held to be clearly seperable.

(3) Important features of the day hospital result from the fact that the hospital is itself only one part of a complex system of care for the elderly, involving also other social work, geriatric, psychiatric and medical services (see also Daatland 1982). This point has two implications. The perceptions of groups outside the hospital (including relatives) have an important bearing upon its operation and the terms in which it should be evaluated. Additionally, there is a methodological dilemma. A case study approach to the research is the only way to achieve the depth of detailed investigation that is clearly required to reach the research objectives. Yet the case study tends to restrict the view of the institution as a part of a wider system.

In the next chapter we turn to this and other methodological issues as we describe the design of the study and our methods of data collection.

CHAPTER THREE

Study Design and Data Collection

Introduction

In this chapter we first describe the development of the study and the evolution of the research problem. Second, we detail our data sources and methods of data collection. Third, we outline briefly some general issues of research methodology that arose during the course of the project and are likely to recur in similar work.

Developing the study

From the start our project had a dual focus. By describing the way in which one new hospital was operating, the research sought to contribute to our understanding of the nature and development of psychogeriatric day hospital services. Through this description the research also aimed to explore the problems of embarking upon evaluative research in this field. Slightly elaborated then, the two research objectives could be described as:

(1) to provide an account of the services of a new psychogeriatric day hospital and suggest what factors were most influential on the course of this development; and
(2) to explore some of the conceptual and methodological problems of evaluating new health services with particular reference to 'defining objectives', 'measuring outcomes' and 'determining criteria of success'. This second aim would entail describing the different purposes of the hospital, held and acted upon, by different groups, at different times, in different contexts, for different reasons and with different effects. It was a basic premise of the research that without the empirical study of these differences any attempt to evaluate a service

the nature of which had not been established, on the basis of criteria the relevance of which was debatable, would have been entirely premature.

These, then, were the project's aims. However, they had not been simply forged. The plans for the research upon which data collection was based were developed over several months and were the outcome of discussions between various parties to the research enterprise; civil servants, health administrators, medical professionals and other academics as well as the research workers themselves. We refer to these discussions both because the activities of launching and commissioning a project have an important bearing upon the design of evaluative research and because this project has much in common with other evaluative studies in this respect (cf. Becker 1970, part I; Bulmer ed. 1978, part I; Bulmer 1982; Stevenson 1983).

First there was the original suggestion for the project. In the autumn of 1979 a community medicine specialist in a Scottish health board responded to the funding body's publicly expressed interest in 'naturally occuring experiments' in the health service, by indicating considerable local interest in the evaluation of a new psychogeriatric day hospital which was opening shortly. The senior author then began to explore the possibilities for an evaluative study, visiting the hospital and health board offices and preparing a discussion note which served as the basis for a small grant in support of preliminary research. Thus, although strictly speaking the project was not a commissioned piece of work since it was supported as the result of a research proposal from a grant applicant to a funding body, it did arise in part at the initiative of the relevant health board and through discussions between representatives of the health board and a government agency. These initiatives were largely responsible for the timing of the research, its location and the research problem in embryonic form.

Throughout the early negotiations a number of points emerged as important. There was a sense of urgency; the research should start as soon as possible. Otherwise there seemed little point in having selected a new hospital in the first place. Ideally the research would have started before the hospital opened. This is often the case with evaluative studies. The designs that first come to mind often require the research to be established in advance of the service being evaluated (see, e.g., Weiss 1972, ch. 4; Sheldon 1984; Goldberg 1984). Yet typically this does not occur and our study design had to cope with this. It was also clear that the hospital might serve a rather wide range of different objectives and any research would need to take account of this as an important part of the hospital's development (for the classic study, see Perrow 1963). This, too, is typical of new organizations. Finally, because of both practical and methodological difficulties, it was evident that the controls of an experiment or clinical trial were quite out of the question (cf. Cochrane 1972 with Illsley 1980). Thus the research would have to find other ways of 'evaluating' the service and any such study was bound to differ substantially from a traditional piece of evaluative research. Much evaluative research appears to encounter these difficulties yet they are not always confronted face on.

There was also a further problem. In general, practitioners and administrators saw evaluation as, in principle, a straightforward exercise. A research project would simply collect the data and deal with technical complications that might arise through data collection and analysis. Support for evaluation which did not approach the task in this way was muted on several counts. Our study design, which tried to take seriously the issues in evaluative research which we have raised in Chapter 1, was seen as introducing unnecessary complications. There was a straightforward question – 'Has the impact of this day hospital upon the community proved beneficial?' – and what was thought to be required was research which would just measure that. The study was seen as failing to specify any 'outcome' measures or what objectives of the hospital were to be evaluated and how. In general it was felt that the study did not fit that rational model of research which the term 'evaluation' tended to suggest (cf. McGrew et al., eds., 1982).

Thus in preparing the design for the main phase of the project we learned that a particular mode of health service 'evaluation' is so deeply embedded in administrative and professional (and some academic) practice that any study which departs from this mode has to treat the term 'evaluation' with considerable caution. So inasmuch as 'evaluative' research rests on a presumed rational relationship between means and ends in service provision and on a requirement to specify in advance of the research the service objectives, etc., then this study was not an 'evaluative' study but rather a study of some of the problems associated with evaluative research. That is why the distinction is drawn throughout this research between 'topic' and 'resource' (Zimmerman and Pollner 1971). The objectives, etc., of the day hospital were seen, at least initially, as topics for research investigation rather than as resources to be defined in advance and used as tools for research.

As a new psychogeriatric day hospital, the particular hospital suggested for the research proved to be an especially good location for this type of study. First, it was a new organization and it was possible for the research to take advantage of that. Of course, few organizations are entirely stable over time and, as historical studies of hospitals have shown, the goals, objectives and influences of different groups are continually altering (Werry et al. 1974). However, change in the early months is often particularly clear and, most important for our purposes, debate and conflict about hospital objectives was often quite explicit at that time and thus most readily observable. So research attention was drawn to issues which might otherwise have passed unnoticed. Second, the activities of diagnosis and prognosis in geriatric psychiatry are sufficiently flexible (Copeland et al. 1975; Isaacs and Post eds. 1978; Marsden 1978; Ron et al. 1979) to allow for an especially clear expression of a wide range of interpretations – on the part of nursing staff, paramedicals, social workers, relatives and others – of the nature of the problem as well as the nature of a suitable solution. Perceptions of the services of this kind of hospital were therefore particularly charaterized by divergence and ambiguity. Third, as we have noted in Chapter 2, the hospital involved a wide range of different kinds of staff with social work services playing a more significant role in this hospital than is usual within the health service.

As we entered the main phase of the project, the aims of the research, stated earlier briefly, could be spelled out a little in the form of a series of questions. Thus:

(1) What were the different and significant groups involved in the operation of the day hospital? Initial study suggested, at least, the following list: consultant psychiatrist, day hospital nurses, ward nursing staff, social worker, area team social workers, residential social workers, community nurse, occupational therapist, chiropodist, physiotherapist, medical nurse, home-help organizers, general practitioners, relatives, patients and hospital administrators. Of course, these groups varied in significance and, within the research resources available to us, we did not expect to be able to give full attention to them all.
(2) What were their conceptions of the objectives of the hospital, of relevant measures of the outcomes of its services and of criteria for judging success?
(3) In what ways did the different groups implement these objectives as they saw them in the part that they played in the hospital. How did this process, in turn, influence their conceptions of the hospital's services and the problems of its patients?
(4) What factors might explain why the hospital was viewed in particular and different ways?
(5) What were the implications of such an analysis of the hospital for the way in which evaluative research should be conducted?

These questions formulate the evaluative problem somewhat differently from the way in which it is posed in much of the research literature. We discussed that point in Chapter 1. They also embody three presumptions which were not entirely shared by those with whom we negotiated the research plans: first, that a 'controlled experiment' is not possible (even if it were desirable); second, that there are a range of views about the right criteria of 'success'; third, that the nature of the service to be evaluated often remains, initially, unestablished. Our task was to launch an evaluative study in health care consistent with these starting points.

Throughout the development of this research there was one further feature of setting up the study that seemed to be important. Although, as we have described, it was necessary to negotiate the nature of the evaluative exercise with professionals, administrators and others, seldom was any doubt expressed about the desirability of 'evaluation' as a basic feature of health service provision. Neither were practical or ethical objections raised to data collection, in spite of a certain amount of intrusion which some of the methods entailed. This respect for the activity of 'evaluation' underlined the importance of being very clear indeed about the nature of the social process in which we were engaging as we undertook that kind of research.

Data collection

Data collection was divided into three phases. The first phase was a short feasibility study. The second phase involved approximately three months' pilot work spread mainly through the spring and summer of 1980 and the preparation of a full grant application and research design. Finally, the main study was conducted over the two-year period 1981–2. We can use these headings to organize an account of the data that we collected although, of course, in several respects, and for several reasons (see Douglas 1976) matters were not quite as neat as these headings imply.

First, in practice the distinction between pilot and main stage data softened as the project progressed. In the chapters that follow we often draw upon the pilot field notes and present extracts alongside main stage data. One set of interviews initially intended to provide only exploratory background information actually yielded data of much greater importance. Also some of what we thought were only preliminary observations held firm. On the other hand some of the main stage data which we expected to be significant turned out to be less revealing than we had anticipated and some tentative and exploratory work continued on the study right up to the termination of the research.

Second, we deliberately maintained a flexible approach because the institution that we were studying was, especially at first, changing quite rapidly. The best example of this was data collected on the relatives' support group. This group was not created until some months after the start of the research. It therefore played no part in the feasability investigation although it was eventually a most important source of data in our study of the relatives' perspective on the services.

Third, any neat plans for separate stages of data collection also become confused by the requirements of free movement between theory and data which good research design entails (Glaser and Strauss 1967). Chapter 1 of this book was not, of course, written first. Since we learned as we progressed, and since our design reflects a theory of evaluation, there was continual interaction between data collection, research design and the project's theoretical stance.

Finally, as Johnson (1975) has demonstrated, most research is much more confused in practice than the subsequent published accounts tend to imply. Although we try here to present as accurate a picture as possible of the way in which the project developed, both the constraints of academic convention and the tendency to impose order in social life where there is none (Berger and Luckmann 1967) probably produce a picture of a project which fails to do justice to its incremental and disjointed character. There is no reason to suppose that the process of planning and developing a research project is any more 'rational' than the process of planning and developing the hospital services that we are evaluating (Hammond 1964; Bell and Newby, eds. 1977).

Nevertheless, with these reservations in mind, we can use the three broad phases of the research to organize our comments.

Feasibility study

This phase of the research was brief and was intended simply to establish whether or not it would be sensible to contemplate evaluative research in this setting. We visited the hospital, and were shown around it like any other of the many officials who were visiting it during its early weeks. We met the sister-in-charge and social worker and discussed the possibility of evaluative research with them. We visited the health board offices, discussed the proposal with the officials most concerned and consulted the most important of the planning papers. We also conducted a preliminary review of the literature on research directly related to the functioning of psychogeriatric day hospitals. This review suggested that topics dealt with included: problems of the excessive demand for hospital beds and the silting up of day-care facilities, the interrelationship between social and medical problems of patients, the comparison of community with hospital care as measured by follow-up studies, the interrelationship between services and the roles and attitudes of relatives towards the mentally disturbed elderly. (We shall refer to this literature where relevant in subsequent chapters.) It was clear that, with some exceptions (e.g. Page 1976; Platt et al. 1980), the major issues of evaluative research which we had begun to identify had not received the attention that they warranted.

On the basis of this work we concluded that:

(1) it would be practicable to mount a study of the hospital;
(2) access to the necessary data would present no major problems;
(3) an evaluative study would have a place in the literature; and
(4) the 'traditional' mode of evaluative research seemed not to cope with some features of the service.

We then prepared a discussion note which served as the basis for a small grant in support of the pilot study.

Pilot study

The pilot study represented some three month's work spread over a twelve-month period. During this time we collected data through the following activities.

(1) We reviewed health board papers on the design and planning of the hospital in much greater detail than we had done previously. We paid particular attention to the minutes of a working party which had been responsible for this planning, together with associated correspondence between area and district administrators. We copied and made notes on these documents.
(2) We began to attend the meetings of the working party, which also assumed responsibility for the evaluation of the hospital's services as they developed. Principally we adopted observer status but contributed to discussion when evaluation was considered.
(3) We began to attend the weekly staff meetings at the hospital. Here we adhered strictly to observer status.
(4) We undertook participant observation at the regular meetings of the relatives' group, which was established during this period. Here we adopted a position close to the 'observer' end of the participant observer continuum.
(5) We reviewed case notes on the population of hospital patients.

Throughout this phase we recorded our observations, conversations, impressions and tentative conclusions in dictated field notes which were transcribed onto several hundred pages of typescript. We consulted these notes repeatedly during the rest of the research.

By the time that pilot work was finished we had completed several tasks. We had developed good working relationships with hospital staff and established the level of co-operation which the main study would require (cf. Johnson 1975, chs. 3 and 4). We had thoroughly explored the feasibility of a range of data-collecting techniques in the context of this hospital and established that later plans were practicable. We had piloted different styles of interviewing. We knew what raw data was to hand, what data would have to be more actively created, how long data collection of various kinds would take, how frequently meetings took place and many of the other details upon which the accurate and successful planning, costing and execution of fieldwork depends.

We had also learned a good deal about the work of the hospital. For example, we had a picture of the kind of patients who were admitted, how long they stayed, whether they were discharged and how this decision was taken. We gained some idea of the part played in the life of the hospital by different professional groups and how they linked together. We knew something of the way in which relatives were involved in the care of patients. We could describe arrangements for transporting patients to and from the hospital.

But even more important than these first findings, we had established numerous working hypotheses to guide the collection of further data. For example we took a provisional view of the main function of the relatives' group. We developed a view about how 'patient flow' would be maintained. Tentatively, we outlined a theory of the role of the idea of 'success' within the culture of the hospital. Much data collection in the main stage of the project was geared towards testing these hypotheses - or provisional conclusions - and suggesting alternative accounts if they proved to be deficient.

On the basis of this pilot work we prepared a full research design and grant application (which was successful) in support of the major study. The principal researcher was joined by two research assistants and a part-time secretary and the main phase of data collection then took place over a period of two years.

The main stage of data collection

The main stage of the project entailed data collection of several different kinds: the analysis of hospital records, field notes on observations and conversations, transcribed recordings of meetings involving staff and relatives, and interviews with staff and relatives. At points in the research we depend quite heavily upon the interview data although, as at earlier stages in the project, wherever possible we prefer to rely upon 'naturally occurring' materials (see Denzin 1978a).

(1) INTERVIEWS We interviewed two sets of respondents. First we conducted sixteen interviews with those health board officials, specialist advisers, medical professionals, nurses and other workers concerned with the planning and operation of the hospital. Initially we intended to interview just a very small number

of 'key informants' to provide limited background information. However it was quickly apparent that by extending the interviews and transcribing them completely they would yield more substantial data than originally anticipated. The sixteen respondents included area, district and hospital administrators, nursing and community medicine specialists, nursing officers, the sister-in-charge, a senior enrolled nurse, the medical officer (who was also a local GP), a consultant, social worker, a community nurse and ward sisters in Park Hospital.

Each of the interviews lasted about an hour. They varied between a half and one-and-three-quarter hours. Each was tape recorded and transcribed. They were semi-structured, each covering the same broad issues but varying in detail depending upon the position, knowledge and interests of respondents in order to achieve equivalence at the level of meaning. (For the classic statement of this problem, see Benney and Hughes 1956.) The topics covered included respondents' views on the aims of the day hospital, the degree of 'success' that it was achieving, the basis on which this judgement was made and the respondents' own experience of being involved in the new development. We also asked respondents for their views on the future development of the hospital. The general style of interviewing involved a good deal of probing, asking respondents to explain and elaborate upon their replies. Although we asked them directly about the success of the hospital and how they measured it, statements about assessment criteria often emerged most clearly in discussions of particular aspects of the development and operation of the hospital.

Although all our data are presented under the usual conventions of research about the anonymity of research subjects, in presenting material from these interviews we have been particularly careful to alter unimportant details to make sure that individuals cannot be identified.

Second, we interviewed a sample of patients' relatives. Starting from a randomly selected date around half way through the main stage of the project, we selected the first twenty-five 'suitable' cases referred to the hospital. 'Suitable' cases were those in which at least one relative was in regular contact with the patient and playing some part in their care. These cases were identified by inspecting the minutes of Tuesday meetings which recorded all referrals and then consulting the social worker about the position of any relatives. In arranging the interviews we contacted just one relative, as is the practice in most studies of carers (e.g. Sanford 1975; Gilliard and Watt 1982; Allen et. al., 1983b; Charlesworth et al. 1984). But since it became clear that the notion of a single 'primary carer' did not fit many of the circumstances that we encountered, in several cases the interview was conducted with two or more respondents. Our objective was to interview relatives twice – at patient admission and then at discharge. In seventeen cases the relatives were interviewed twice – first at admission, and then either at discharge or after between two and a half and six months if the patient had not been discharged when the time came to complete our interviewing programme nine months after the date on which we started it. The relatives in the remaining eight cases were interviewed only once either because the patient did not attend at all (two cases) or only briefly (six cases).

These interviews were again semi-structured, tape recorded and transcribed.

We asked relatives about their perceptions of the patient's problem and their experience of receiving services, generally and in connection with the day hospital in particular.

We did not interview patients in any formal way. We do not rule out the possibility of such interviews in this kind of research but we concluded that collecting and analysing such data raised issues which were beyond the scope and resources of this particular project. Although we had some informal conversations with patients during the course of our fieldwork, our access to a 'consumer perspective' is principally through the interviews with relatives.

(2) HOSPITAL RECORDS We collected and studied the hospital records on two samples of cases. Information was extracted from the card index and from case files. (We have described the records system in the hospital in greater detail in Chapter 2.) The first sample included all 103 cases admitted to the hospital over the first fourteen months of its operation. Because the hospital began from a zero base, we took this period in order to give an early approximation to a normal twelve months. The second sample entailed prospective data collection on all forty-five patients admitted during a six-month period in the middle of the main stage of the project, with records information consulted over a three-month follow-up period. We also collected information on all eighteen cases referred and considered for a day hospital place but not admitted during the six months. We hoped that by taking a prospective sample we would be able to triangulate data on these patients with data that we were collecting elsewhere at the same time (Denzin 1978; Denzin, ed. 1978b, part XII). We also consulted the records of the twenty-six cases which were discussed at the Tuesday meetings during the six-month period, but not as 'referrals' to the day hospital. (These patients were discussed because they were of interest to staff attending the meeting and because it was hoped that patients would move between the day hospital and in-patient beds.) On some of these cases the information available was limited.

Data extracted from records included such information as dates of referral, admission and discharge, reasons given for admission and discharge, diagnosis, Crichton ratings, next of kin, medical treatment and destination on discharge. We also collected, verbatim, substantial material from nursing notes and medical officer reports and especially from the psychiatric domiciliary visit reports and social worker's background reports.

We used material from these two samples to assemble a statistical account of referrals, attendance patterns at the hospital and discharges over a period of time. These samples are also the main source of qualitative data taken from records used throughout the study.

(3) OBSERVATIONS OF MEETINGS We attended many of the weekly Tuesday meetings during this period of fieldwork and the majority of the meetings of the relatives' group over a period of eighteen months. We dictated field notes, which were transcribed, of these meetings. These notes recorded our observations and included short sections of the discussion verbatim. Some of these fieldnotes also

assumed the status of preliminary working papers as we began to analyse and interpret our observations in the light of the emerging research questions. As at the pilot stage, we adhered to observer status in the Tuesday meetings but were occasionally marginal participants at the relatives' group.

(4) RECORDED MEETINGS We tape recorded a number of the Tuesday meetings and meetings of the relatives' group. Staff were initially reluctant to admit a tape recorder to the Tuesday meetings but then agreed to it after discussion of the potential value of these data. Staff also initially felt that the presence of a recorder would inhibit relatives at the relatives' group although relatives themselves raised no objections, saying that they expected such an activity to be a part of a research project. Although transcribing these tapes was complicated and time consuming, we completed full typed transcripts of four Tuesday meetings and four relatives' groups. We introduced the recorder several meetings prior to those selected for transcription and we know, from our previous observations of both kinds of meetings, that any short-term effect of the presence of a small recorder quickly faded. These direct recordings allow us to present lengthy verbatim extracts from the discussions.

(5) GENERAL OBSERVATIONS Throughout the entire period of the study we also made general observations on the life of the day hospital. We conversed with patients, accompanied nursing auxiliaries on the coach journeys to and from patients' homes, joined in some of the ward activities and other aspects of the social life of the hospital, spoke with the domestic and junior nursing staff and observed nurses' treatment of patients and their dealings with relatives when they visited the hospital. We kept a record of our activities through the research, recording our further impressions, conversations and observations as we had done during pilot work. As with other materials these notes were taped, transcribed and filed under the headings that began to emerge as the framework for organizing our material.

Conclusion

With the framework of ideas for a pluralistic evaluation of the day hospital in mind, this chapter (apart from the short introduction) has so far been divided into two sections. The first described the way in which the initial evaluative issue developed into a set of specific research questions. The second has described in detail the data that we collected and the way we collected them. Our emphasis upon pluralistic evaluation is generally reflected in our attempts to tap as many perspectives as possible through as many data sources as possible using as wide a variety of methods as possible in order to maximize the 'rich' quality of the materials upon which the subsequent conclusions in this book are based. Many of the research issues which we have touched upon through this chapter have been very fully discussed in the research literature, particularly under the headings of 'participant observation' or 'qualitative research' (e.g. Becker 1958; Selltiz et al. 1966; Lofland 1971; Bulmer ed 1977; see also Phillips 1973 and Knapp

1981). Nevertheless it is instructive to mention one or two issues which were of special concern in this particular study.

Our research design presumed a team of research workers (cf. Douglas 1976). In part, a team was necessary because of the volume of data that we needed to collect in a comparatively short time. It was also necessary because, in pursuit of collecting data from varied sources, we sometimes needed to collect data in different places at the same time. There were also a limited number of occasions, for example in observing complicated meetings, on which the presence of two research workers concentrating on different facets of events was valuable.

Even with a team of research workers there is the issue of establishing the boundaries for such a study and establishing criteria for data exclusion. We had initially expected to interview GPs, social workers in residential accommodation and other professional groups who had contact, through the system of health and welfare care for the elderly mentally infirm, with the day hospital. In practice the day hospital had contacts with many more professionals in each of these various groups than we had initially expected. For example, the population of the day hospital covered a large number of GPs and few GPs had more than one or two patients at the hospital. The size of the sample of respondents that we would have needed to interview in order to collect, for example, material on GPs' attitudes would therefore have had to have been more extensive than our resources allowed. There are points in the research where the absence of data on GP attitudes and perspectives, in particular, is something which we regret. Nevertheless, we realized in considering these issues that further activities would have taken us into a study of the overall system of care for the elderly mentally infirm which we were not equipped to conduct.

The issues of qualitative as opposed to quantitative data collection methods feature in much research literature (see, e.g., Irvine et al., eds. 1979, especially chapter 1). We have regarded any debate of qualitative *versus* quantitative methods as artificial. All data is potentially biased and the research design must guard against that. When we have been able to quantify precisely, we have done so. But frequently a qualitative account, for example of the events at a meeting, must precede any attempt at the quantification of variables and much of the research was designed to isolated those factors which are important, prior to their subsequent and more precise measurement.

There is also the issue of how to *manage* large amounts of qualitative data (Blaxter, ed. 1979). Our methods generated a considerable volume of typescript of interviews, transcripts of meetings and field notes. The magnitude of the task of producing and indexing these materials led us to restrict the transcription of direct tape recordings. Shorter field notes tend to advance the analysis although they may lose some of the raw data.

Finally, Denzin (1978a) has long advocated the triangulation of data in research methods. The view that a conclusion is much stronger when supported by data from different sources was a view which we accepted in designing this research. Because we interviewed as many different groups as possible, inspected hospital records, made transcripts of discussions and meetings, and took field notes on observations and conversations, we can approach most topics from several perspectives. Thus, for example, on the subject of the place of relatives in the hospital we can consult data from transcripts and from field notes on group meetings, from staff discussions about particular relatives at Tuesday meetings, from staff responses in interviews on the subject, from interviews with relatives, and from hospital records on the patients in question.

Individually our data sets have significant weaknesses. Taken together, however, we argue that they possess very considerable strengths.

CHAPTER FOUR

The Meanings of Success

Introduction

In previous chapters we have seen that a key feature in evaluative research is the way in which the selection of criteria for assessing service performance is undertaken. As Schwartz and Alwin (1971, p. 632) comment:

> The development of criteria of success ... is in itself a singularly difficult issue ... But the clear development of the criteria of success of any program and the operationalization of these criteria are the preconditions for conducting any evaluative research, and it is precisely here that all other problems meet; the problem of theoretical and ideological differences, the problem of professional quarreling, the problem of auspices under which the research is conducted, the problem of trying to maintain one's own professional integrity, and the problem of trying to develop rigorous designs. All of these meet in the problem of criteria development.

Our approach to the problem is to adopt a pluralistic stance and set out the *several* meanings of success, as defined by those responsible for planning, implementing and using the service.

In this chapter, therefore, we set out the several ways in which patients, relatives and staff involved in the planning and operation of the day hospital define its success. As we have described in Chapter 3, we conducted a set of semi-structured, tape recorded interviews with relevant staff in which, amongst other matters, we asked them about the success of the hospital, what they considered to be relevant measures of success and how they felt that the hospital was performing, and was intended to perform, on these counts. We also interviewed a sample of patients' relatives.

It is important to stress that this chapter documents the perspectives of members of the organization, as recorded in our interviews. Accordingly we shall, through the rest of the chapter, quote fully from these interviews. We shall describe six separate meanings of success. These provide the criteria, from within the system of care, for use by staff in presenting their work as successful and by staff and relatives in assessing the performance of the institution as a whole. These criteria also form the framework for the rest of our research and we shall consider each in some detail.

At this stage our account is merely descriptive in the sense that we simply lay out these interpretations as a framework for subsequent analysis. We are not yet attempting to rank the criteria in any order of importance or describe their practical impact. As we shall show, some are especially important within the culture of the institution and some are more dominant than others in shaping the operation of the hospital. Some groups of staff and relatives employ some criteria and some others. Some employ several criteria and some adopt a more single-minded stance. There is also variation depending upon the situational constraints under which staff are operating and upon variations in the requirement to demonstrate success in their own work. In practice different criteria are used in different ways by different groups at different times in different contexts for different purposes with different effects. We shall turn to these variations in subsequent chapters and we shall need to add much additional data to the interview material which we present here. But the first task is to describe what the different criteria are.

Six criteria of success

At least six separate ways in which 'success' for this day hospital is given meaning – and thus the hospital's objectives and desirable modes of operation are specified – emerge from the interviews with staff and relatives. We describe these as:

(1) success meaning free patient flow;
(2) success meaning clinical cure for patients;
(3) success meaning the provision of an integrated service;
(4) success meaning beneficial impact on related services;
(5) success meaning support for relatives; and
(6) success meaning service of high quality.

Patient flow

The first refers to the 'flow' of patients through the system of referral, admission, treatment and discharge, into and out of the day hospital and related institutions. Thus, as it was reported to us, the hospital should reduce demand for in-patient beds:

> Well the main achievement is to keep the elderly as fit and as able as we can in the community and to stop – try and reduce the demand on in-patient beds and to prevent people coming into beds prematurely and keep the patient in the community as long as we can.
>
> (*A nurse*)

This, in turn, should shorten waiting lists for these beds:

> We have a large waiting list of psychogeriatric patients waiting on admission and we have nothing in the foreseeable future to offer them in the way of beds other than hoping beds we have already becoming available in ones and two...
>
> (*A community nurse*)

> I was led to believe that the whole purpose of the day hospital ... was because of the waiting list for places which we did not have for psychogeriatrics...
>
> (*A nursing officer*)

The day hospital should prevent and delay admission of patients to in-patient beds.

> ... we find that we're getting far too many patients in who should be in the community and hopefully the day hospital is going to stop them coming in at an early stage and the longer we can keep people in the community the better it's going to be for themselves and the health service as a whole.
>
> (*An administrator*)

Moreover it should facilitate the discharge of patients from Park Hospital:

> My hopes right from the start would be where there was slack was that we might have had some other in-patients, perhaps the cream of the in-patients who had potential for discharge, having an opportunity to have the benefits of an intensive sort of treatment regime...
>
> (*A nursing officer*)

and it should improve the use of particular categories of beds by the correct categories of patients;

> ... it was hoped that the selection of patients would be such that there would be patients that we could do something for – hm – it's very easy to take the first ten people that come along, you have to be selective ... there is no point in filling the place and then you can't admit somebody else who could benefit ... The person who gets most benefit should be the person who would get the ... place; there should be a turnover of about sixty or seventy a year.
>
> (*A consultant*)

> I think the main thing in [the day hospital] is now that ... most of the psychogeriatric population who've got a psychiatric problem are coming through [the day hospital], we're getting people into the right places that they should be ... I think we're routeing them the right way now. I think eventually – they are having a – y'know an effect on the in-patient population. The right people are getting in, put it that way.
>
> (*A nursing sister*)

The free flow of patients is also held to be important in the context of the pathways which patients follow through the overall system of care. Thus the day hospital should more efficiently mesh in patient referral to health service psychogeriatric care with other services:

> We're accommodating many people and many services.
>
> (*A social worker*)

> Y'see another point is that when a referral comes [here] not all these patients are ... admitted ... It quite often turns out that [the social worker] is able to arrange some other kind of help, such as somebody going for day care in one of the residential units or even exceptionally going into an eventide home,—so that - hm - apart from the places we have here, the team—is - hm - really functioning on a wider basis.
>
> (*A psychiatrist*)

Above all, the innovation should avoid 'silting up' both in the day hospital itself and in other parts of the hospital system to which it relates:

> It's rather nice to have some coming in and some going out.
>
> (*A nursing officer*)

> You have to be very much aware of the need to - hm - keep some sort of flow through the day hospital and not allow it simply to fill up with demented people ... I think the main things I was concerned about in the very beginning were the possibility that it might fill up with people [where] there was really no progress, or very little progress, and that you would get to a stage comparable to the one with the psychogeriatric beds where we're just full up and y'know people went on a waiting list and so on, that's what I've been afraid of all along.
>
> (*A psychiatrist*)

> We thought that if [the day hospital] was going to be effective at all and relieve a great many families, then there would have to be a throughput, patients would have to be in and out...
>
> (*A nursing administrator*)

> Well there's always a waiting - there's always a big - when one stops there are always other ones to fill the gap. I mean to say - that as long as they still take him - I'm quite pleased an' that.
>
> (*A relative*)

So overall, there is widespread accord amongst our respondents with the general rubric that the day hospital should (in the words of a nursing officer) 'provide us with a stepping stone, both from the community into the hospital and from the hospital into the community'.

Clinical cure

A second, and perhaps the most obvious, criterion refers to the success of the hospital in improving the clinical condition of patients eligible for admission.

> We appreciate everything that's being done. Our biggest concern is if we just could see a big improvement in her. But the doctor said right enough, it would be slow.
>
> (*A relative*)

Such a perspective, reflecting a 'disease model' of psychiatric practice, views the conditions from which patients are suffering as akin to other kinds of medical illness and likewise amenable to treatment and cure. The importance of showing improvement on measurement scales such as the Crichton scale, which are used to assess patients as a part of the hospital's regular nursing programme, features particularly in accounts of the use of this criterion. As one respondent explained:

> It was hoped that there would be a *clear measurement* of [the patients'] clinical situation, so that you could get some sort of scale as to whether they were making progress or they weren't. This is the whole idea of this Crichton scale and so on, so that we can begin to *measure* the patients' response to treatment, to medication and so on, and to see whether in fact they're coping...
>
> (*An administrator*)

A nurse explained the practicalities of this ideal:

> ... We do it [test patients] every week and, if the care plan is working out, that scaling rate should come down and hopefully we try to get them down to eleven which we will do. That means that the patient can be totally maintained in the community on their own ... if they're at that for a month or so then that ... [whistles] their physical and mental state is being maintained and that patient is ready to be tried in the community on their own and that's why ... we bring it to the case conference then.
>
> (*A senior nurse*)

Nevertheless the imprecision of clinical judgements in this field are recognized and this particular criterion is not advanced without some considerable reservation.

> ... This is where it is very difficult, when you are talking about clinical outcomes and that, and doctors would be very jealously guarding their position – you can't dictate in ... precise terms, exactly what y'know, ... is going to be – hm – y'know – there's just this general feeling that the day hospital would bring some relief...
>
> (*An administrator*)

This difficulty means that although the clinical efficacy of the hospital's treatment programme may well be the most obvious criterion for measuring its success, in practice, as we shall see, in many situations staff resort to other measures.

Integrated service

The third criterion for considering the success of the hospital refers to the effective integration of services both within the day hospital and between the hospital and related institutions. Great value is attached to good communication, good external communications being particularly important in co-ordination of day hospital services with other services with which it has links. Emphasis is also placed on co-ordination and co-operation between the several professions involved directly in patient care. Furthermore the organization of the day hospital should encourage staff to derive maximum job satisfaction and work together effectively as an integrated team.

The development of co-ordination between the day hospital and community-based services, both medical and social work, is especially important in these terms:

> We're getting a greater liaison going with all the services, that it's not nearly as hard now when you phone up for a GP, or a home help or a clinic or a health visitor, they know through the centre, through the day hospital, what we're after and how much we can help and how much they can help us. I think ... it's a focal point to bring all the services together...
>
> (*A community nurse*)

I think that the only way, the only way that both social work *and* health service can deal with problems such as this ... that a combination of the services is the only way things will work. That it *requires* the administration to *understand* what you're trying to do, and it *requires* them to *provide* what is necessary.

(*A social worker*)

Certainly close organizational links developed between the day hospital and Park Hospital in arrangements for both administrative matters and the interchange of patients and the ideal of collaboration between the two institutions is significant in considering the day hospital to be successful through the organization and integration of its services.

... It's interesting to note that we didn't really think much about the proximity of the wards when this [the day hospital] was planned, and in fact it turned out to be a very valuable thing, perhaps one of the things that we didn't plan which has come off very well by accident, having the wards adjacent to the day hospital...

(*A community medicine specialist*)

... in the early stages I had a very open mind about this, and I did not immediately say the day hospital should be situated in the grounds of Park Hospital. Now that I know how the collaboration has built up between the wards and the day hospital I'm greatly relieved that we did not choose any of these other sites, because although in theory the machinery would have been there, in practice it would have been very much more difficult ...

(*A psychiatrist*)

This integration of services is also considered to be important because it is accompanied by integrated professional work leading to good teamwork within the hospital.

... There's the development of the team which is all important in my opinion, which I think is developed - eh - very, very well indeed, and I think that it is still developing.

(*A social worker*)

And team work, in turn, makes a major contribution to maintaining staff morale in an area of practice which is often considered to be uninteresting and of low status:

You must remember that apart from this particular unit, working in psychogeriatrics can be a pretty dull business and largely custodial care...

(*A commonity medicine specialist*)

... and I think that ... that there is this need for a little flag-waving as well which will have a very direct bearing on the people...

(*The same specialist*)

... and the staff themselves I think have - hm - look on it as something special and this being the case I'm quite sure that this, passes on, this feeling passes on to the patients themselves. But we just feel we're special, so we try to give of our best and it ends up something special.

(*A nursing officer*)

Hm – there's a satisfaction in it being a new venture ... and I've found this has helped *my* morale. In the Health Service just now morale is a very important point ... it seems to be cutbacks rather than development at the present time but here there has been an island of development...

(*A psychiatrist*)

Hm – I suppose the morale of the team has been all important.

(*A consultant*)

I think that perhaps is one of the values of a place like this, that both the staff involved and those who are on the fringe of it feel they are doing something...

(*A community medicine specialist*)

In the context of ... [this area] the work that is being done at [the day hospital] is – interesting work ... now I think that applies to all of the professions because the work there is ... being done in a stimulating environment ... hm – ... there's very much team spirit operating...

(*An administrator*)

Impact on related services

The fourth criterion that emerged from our interviews is also related to the way in which the system of care is organized. This criterion of success refers to the evaluation of the day hospital in terms of the contribution that it makes to related services. Such a view dictates that we examine the day hospital as one component of an overall system of health and social care for the elderly mentally infirm. Even if the hospital has no significant and demonstrable direct effect on the elderly, it may nevertheless be justified in the help it offers to social workers, GPs, district nurses, the home-help service, or whatever. Respondents commented upon the way in which they saw the day hospital assisting GPs who could now refer patients with some hope of admission; consultant geriatricians who could refer on their elderly psychiatric cases; the consultant psychiatrists who now saw some hope of relieving demand on beds; and social workers and others in 'community' services who were offered help with their most difficult cases. One respondent gave an example:

INTERVIEWER: 'How would you describe the service that the day hospital is offering to the patients and their families...?'

RESPONDENT: 'Well – one – we offer the community an almost immediate service in that we offer relief for – and I'm talking about GPs and that doesn't always happen in other places ... that you get immediate relief. When I talk about immediate relief it can be immediate ... as we did in one particular case that comes to mind, that [the consultant] saw her in the morning ... and she was in the next day. And that's as immediate as it can be, I think. Eh – generally speaking we can *service* somebody if you like, – hm – within two weeks, that's perhaps the quickest ... Now that relieves the doctor, because it takes the pressure off him, it relieves the pressure from the relatives getting onto him about getting something done.'

(*A social worker*)

Another respondent made a more general comment claiming a significant impact for the hospital on relatives, some patients *and* other services:

The relatives are, I think, the ones who get most benefit from it at the moment and, as I say, the depressed patients get a lot of benefit from it. I think we help the services outside as well, the district nursing services, the home-help service as well, because we can give them information. We can relieve some of the work of the district nurses; if we have the patient in here and there's dressings or bathing etc., to be done, we can in some cases take that over. That gives them more time and relieves them as well. We certainly relieve the GP in a lot of cases where he has the hysterical hypochondriacal patients at him all the time, that's taken away because they feel, we seem to take over as long as they've got someone listening to them, someone dealing with their problems, we take over so we relieve a lot in the community, a lot of the services that are in the community . . .

(*A senior nurse*)

The argument is that there is a kind of domino effect. The impact of the day hospital is cumulative as the effect on other services reverberates through the system. In this way the success of the day hospital in terms of its use to allied services is closely related to its success as measured in other ways;

It helped the relatives which was tied up with the pressure – it takes the pressure off the relatives, therefore the relatives take the pressure off the GP and consequently off our consultants and consequently off our bed state.

(*A nurse*)

Relative support

This mention of the relatives of patients leads us to the fifth criterion. Many respondents said that a most significant measure of the day hospital's achievements is the service which it provides to the relatives:

. . . So many of the relatives were just at the end of their tether, they just didn't think they could cope with the patient and they were really – marriages were beginning to crumble and all sorts of things just because of the strain, and I really think the hospital has helped an awful lot of people that way.

(*A secretary*)

I think when relatives get despondent and frustrated and there's no one to turn to, and they're on the waiting list that's all they'll get doing – eh – I think its a very desperate situation to be in and I think this is the biggest area of success that the day hospital has provided as well.

(*A community nurse*)

Oh I thought this was a good idea because it was also giving me a break two days a week and it was letting her get out.

(*A relative*)

There are several ways in which the day hospital may help. By removing the patient from the home for specified periods it provides respite for the relative from the otherwise constant burden of caring.

Well the fact that the relatives have been able to come for a set number of days, that relieves pressure on the relative looking after them at home.

(*A nursing officer*)

. . . it's my feeling that through the day hospital you're – hm – often giving the family some relief just in that that's the number of hours per week that – eh –

they're free to do other things, now of course other agencies can do that too, but they can't do it with all the kinds of patients that we have here...

(*A psychiatrist*)

As well as simply providing some form of custodial care for the patient, the day hospital should also give positive assistance to the relatives in caring for the patient. This is mainly said to be achieved by educating the relatives in how to manage the patient at home more appropriately.

INTERVIEWER: 'What would you say has been the areas in which the day hospital has made the greatest progress?'
RESPONDENT: 'I think undoubtedly – eh – in – eh – education of relatives, there's no question about that...

(*A community nurse*)

... There's an opportunity during [the period that the patient attends the day hospital] to find out – eh – how they should cope with mother or father when they get him out in ... so they can perhaps sit back and look at the situation, what are they doing that we're not doing – eh – what could we do – eh – in addition to what we have been doing – eh – or what should be stopped that we have been doing y'know, this sort of thing...

(*A community nurse*)

As we have mentioned, the day hospital's function in educating relatives is in part achieved through the medium of a relatives' support group which we shall discuss in detail in subsequent chapters. Provision of emotional support and, to some extent, therapy for relatives is also described as an important feature of the relatives' group in particular and the services of the day hospital in general:

We're offering support to relatives I think to ... even to the extent of, I think, of saving somebody's marriage and somebody's family. I think support is a good thing that they're offered, you're offering comfort, help I suppose, sometimes I think its more like eh – throwing somebody a life-line, a lifebelt, y'know, saying, 'Well, look, it might not be the best but its the best we can do'.

(*A social worker*)

One respondent described in more detail how the day hospital fulfils this supportive function:

Supporting is hm – its knowing what the illness is and y'know letting [the relatives] know that we know what they are going through, that if they have any problems at all that they just need to contact the day hospital and if there's anything I can do then I certainly will try my best to do that and support them in that way and make them feel comfortable with the day hospital that they can phone anytime and that no one will shout down the phone and say, 'Sorry, I can't do anything about that'.

(*A nursing sister*)

Others described the part played by the relatives' support group:

... I think [the relatives' group] possibly has helped some relatives to be able to share their problems with people who have the same problems or greater problems. I think it has helped them, and it has helped them to go back home to look after mother and father in a fresh light.

(*A nursing officer*)

> ... [the relatives' group] gives this opportunity to laugh and to cry at times and to express anger, and the second thing is to educate again but in a very gentle educative way, it is not full-scale education, 'You will come here and you will learn,' but its a very gentle process ...
>
> (*A social worker*)

Some respondents even see the day hospital as affording the opportunity of psychiatric treatment itself to the relatives of patients. The relatives' support group has special value in such a therapeutic context.

> ... [the relatives' group] provides a setting where people can abreact, they can talk about their feelings and embarrassment and aggression in a group of people who are all on the same footing and I think this is very valuable ... I'm now sometimes going into a situation in somebody's home where the main problem really is, say, the daughter's feelings about her dementing mother or father where I almost feel that they don't really need to take the patient on but I'd like to take the relatives. I don't think we have ever really divorced the two things completely ... now I think – hm – eh – someone like this is being often helped through the relatives' group, so that, I think, is a very valuable part of the day hospital.
>
> (*A psychiatrist*)

The facilities and the team of professionals in the day hospital, which work to improve the quality of assessment of patients, should also extend this assessment to the relatives and thus extend the service to the family unit.

> I'm talking not so much from the patient's assessment in the home, but the assessment of the relatives in being able to cope with the individual – eh – and their attitude to do it and their ability to maintain this relative ... and the whole group is being sustained here without any crisis developing but to be able to assess and to be able to read the early warning signs as they appear and to take action before the actual crisis, that is the sort of assessment I'm talking about now ...
>
> (*A community nurse*)

> Certainly there's an awful lot more social implication than what there was at the beginning, y'know we're just building up and we're getting to know, but as we get to know each patient and we get to know each relative, we know exactly what should go into the home and I think becoming more socially oriented as well, than what it was initially. When we came in we were looking at the patient and what we could do for them and now its like treating the family unit, and not treating one person, but treating that one person within that family unit, becoming oriented towards that.
>
> (*A nursing sister*)

Of course assessment and the provision of a psychiatric service to relatives does not automatically advance the interests of the family as this may not accord with the relatives' own perceived needs. We shall return to this point in Chapter 9. The important point here is that – for a significant proportion of staff – the service provided to relatives, particularly through the relatives' group, is central to any consideration of the success of the day hospital.

> ... That's something [the relatives' group] that has really been worthwhile and I think if we are going to say that [the day hospital] has been a success, that's what we've really got to attribute most success to, that area [work with relatives].
>
> (*A community nurse*)

Quality of service

A sixth, and final, criterion for judging the success of the hospital refers to the *quality* of the services. From this perspective the hospital's success may be measured by pointing to a number of features which are desirable *in their own right*. These stand as valuable quite apart from any demonstrable effect on performance measures such as the condition of patients or official admission and discharge statistics. Thus, in summary, the hospital should provide a civilized and caring environment, staff should convey caring attitudes to patients and relatives, and patients should enjoy their time at the hospital.

> It is very nice and very comfortable, it really is. I was amazed the first time I saw it, I mean I expected a sort of bare – I don't know – an institution thing. And it was really completely different from what I thought it would be. I was really amazed when I saw it, I mean there is everything there for their comfort
>
> (*A relative*)

As another respondent explained, the quality of care had featured as a criterion very early in the plans for the hospital:

> The Board's officers were very concerned that the existing vehicles for day care really fell more, without being in any way derogatory, into the sense of being *day centres*, the social services concept. It was questionable to what extent they were carrying out a therapeutic function ... more they were just caring centres ... the day hospital was created to try and inject a new initiative in the care of the elderly and mentally infirm.
>
> (*An administrator*)

And, quite apart from clinical consequences, this initiative had produced results:

> I'm not talking about the clinical side, but the patients seem to be happy. One sat and talked to patients and so on, but whether therapeutically, y'know, it's better or worse than anything else I can't say, but y'know the whole atmosphere it conveys is one of apparent efficiency and friendliness and – y'know, that's something good because you've not got much like that in [this area] y'know, it seems to be stimulating, I think that's something that we're all pleased with.
>
> (*An administrator*)

For the quality of care entailed an improvement in the quality of life:

> I would hope we are rehabilitating them as far as we can and improving their quality of life. I think that's the main thing from – hm – is that the *quality* of life is improved.
>
> (*A senior nurse*)

Conclusion

We began this chapter by recalling a central difficulty in evaluative research. Typically any agreed policies for an institution are stated in only vague and ambiguous terms. As soon as we look for specific statements of aims we usually find that there is a variety of ways in which members define the objectives and success of the service. There is therefore a core problem in research of the development of criteria of success. In this chapter we have reported those criteria of success which are to be found in the day hospital for the elderly mentally infirm which we are studying. In order to avoid either selecting just one of these criteria or of imposing some criterion of our own – we have criticized both options – we are arguing the merits of a pluralistic approach.

Thus these six criteria (see p. 44) will form the framework for analysing and reporting our data. The body of our research report consists of several essays around the six meanings of success. In the final chapter we shall bring together what we consider to be the advantages of this approach to evaluation but we are aware that it has its critics (e.g. Benington 1975) and there is one criticism in particular that should be considered here.

Although a pluralistic evaluation avoids the management (or any other) bias entailed in the selective use of evaluative measures, it may be argued that the emphasis placed upon the way in which members themselves perceive a service, introduces a serious flaw. Such an evaluation can assess a service *only in its own terms*. It is therefore an essentially conservative approach. For defects in a service may well occur because significant groups of professionals, planners, administrators and even consumers are themselves using the wrong criteria to influence the service. Evaluation should be assessing these criteria and thus provide both a radical criticism of the service and suggestions for significant changes and improvements.

The point is undoubtedly an important one (cf. generally, George and Wilding 1976; Taylor-Gooby and Dale 1981; Mishra 1981; Mishra 1984.) but it is a point about the politics of social change rather than the methodology of evaluation research. We have no *a priori* objection to the argument that professionals and others are guided in their actions by inappropriate standards. We do object to the suggestion that the debate about appropriate standards in service provision can be resolved as a technical task at the design stage of evaluation research. It is a debate that has to be resolved on the basis of political, moral and other principles. Of course, there must be a factual basis to the argument and this consists, in part, of information about the standards that guide professionals and others in the operation and use of the service. But this is exactly the kind of data that a pluralistic evaluation produces and that we have presented in this chapter.

Moreover, we do not accept that a pluralistic approach to evaluation is as conservative as it may initially appear. First, its explanatory power is an important aspect of its potential to produce recommendations for change. Second, the approach has, as we have mentioned, considerable advantages when it comes to the implementation of any recommendations. Third, as incrementalists have argued in their analysis of the policy process, policy choices are made from those options which, for a variety of reasons, happen actually to be available. We expect a pluralistic evalutaion to be taken seriously because it operates within the options that are taken seriously by at least some parties to the service. As we have said, debate about adding to that range of options lies outside the realms of evaluative research – not in evaluative research of a supposedly more radical kind. And finally, any limitations that there may be in the scope of the criteria we use in this research are as much a function of limitations in time and other resources at our disposal, as of the approach and methods we pursue. We have explained in Chapter 3 that the more systematic inclusion of GP and residential care perspectives, for example, would have been desirable. We were able to interview relatives. An even more extensive study might include other groups of actors drawn from patients and clients and from the policy-shaping communities of the health, local government and central government sectors. But, whatever the scope of the research, our argument is that a pluralistic evaluation would still be appropriate. That is why we are presenting our analysis of one new service, around six criteria of success, as a worked example of the way in which pluralistic evaluation offers a new direction for evaluative research.

CHAPTER FIVE

Success as Patient Flow

Introduction

In the course of studying staff and relative perceptions of the way in which the hospital should operate, we encountered widespread advocacy in general terms of the importance of 'turnover' in the population of the institution. This concern mirrors the frequent references to 'patient flow' as a criterion for measuring the success of day care for the elderly, which appear in the psychiatric literature (Pathy 1969; Cross et al. 1972; Martin and Millard 1975; Baker and Byrne 1977; Green and Timbury 1979). It is generally felt to be rather obvious that any service claiming to be effective should at least be able to discharge patients regularly and admit new cases. So, throughout the day hospital, there is widespread reference to the 'flow' of patients through the system of referral, admission, treatment and discharge, into and out of the hospital and related institutions, as a basis for organizational practice. 'Patient turnover' is a key evaluative measure.

However, this does not mean that we have in the goal of 'turnover' a simple and self-evident criterion for evaluation. For when we examine in detail how different groups pursue this overall objective, how they perceive the consequences of pursuing it in a variety of ways, and how they adopt particular organizational strategies, we come back to our problem. Much of the hospital's work with patients cannot be understood if we presume that advantage for all lies simply in the shared policy of patients entering and leaving the hospital as rapidly as possible. It very much depends upon just which categories of patients are moving where, how, and with what consequences for what groups of staff, relatives and other patients. There may well be agreement that a day hospital should serve to move patients from the community into in-patient beds and from such beds into the community. But for each group involved in the system of care of which the hospital is part, this perspective yields advantage only when idiosyncratically interpreted. Therefore, as a part of evaluative research, we have to examine the way in which, within the broad consensus, each group perceives and pursues ins own interests in patient turnover.

Constituent interests

We shall consider six constituent groups in the following order: consultants, nurses, general practitioners, social workers, staff of a related hospital (Park Hospital) and patients' relatives.

Consultant psychiatrists

The first of the constituent groups of an institution such as the day hospital is the consultants. Their interest in extending provision for care of psychogeriatric patients throughout the health board area provided much of the original impetus for establishing the day hospital. (Blake 1968; Pathy 1969; Silverman and Val 1975; and Baker and Byrne 1977, have all reported that the role which day hospitals can play in alleviating the demand for in-patient facilities is one of their major contributions.)

The consultants were hopeful that measures would be taken which would have some continuing long-term effect on improving patient flow. Essentially this means, for consultants, that the day hospital should provide them with an additional avenue when considering how to dispose of referrals from GPs. That is the immediate task in hand, described by one consultant psychiatrist thus:

> ... Say as part of my normal duties, maybe my week on call, if I am asked to see an 80-year-old lady within the [day hospital] area, now before, that was a nightmare because you knew very well that the possibility of getting a bed in [the psychiatric hospital] was remote, as it still is, and so there was not really very much you could offer ... First of all I would ask [the social worker] to go and visit and then this may lead to day hospital and to quite a range of things, and believe me that's a great relief ... I know it's made a tremendous difference.

However, more is entailed in successful patient flow for consultants than the hospital simply being an additional referral point. Whereas GPs are primarily interested in the hospital admitting cases, consultants seek also to discharge patients. Goldstein et al. (1968), Irvine (1969) and Pathy (1969), amongst others, have reported a tendency for such day hospitals to 'silt up' because of the difficulties encountered in discharging patients. If the day hospital is to make any contribution to solving the problem of the consultants it must maintain its capacity for channelling patients *to* as well as *from* other parts of the system. Thus, preventing any blockage of patient flow through the day hospital has necessarily become one of the primary concerns of the psychiatrist in charge, a concern which is reflected in the frequent review of occupancy rates at the hospital meetings.

There are several ways in which consultants can attempt to prevent a blockage in the aspects of the system which are of particular concern to them. First, an attempt may be made to control 'bombardment' (the demand for service);

Day Hospt. – impt when considering patient flow.

second, patients may be discharged whenever possible; third, patients may be referred to other services; fourth, there are a variety of arrangements for the use of the hospital in conjunction with in-patients beds. In the context of our present discussion the most interesting feature of them all is the way in which each creates problems for some other group within the system.

(1) CONTROLLING 'BOMBARDMENT' The first way of trying to ensure that the day hospital avoids silt-up is for the consultant psychiatrist to attempt control over the bombardment of referrals from outside sources. A major cost of this strategy is that it conflicts with the interests of GPs and endangers the smooth relations between the hospital and general practice. Since GPs are the major referral agents, this is important. While the day hospital *can* simply refuse further admissions on the grounds of no available places or whatever, constant refusal is obviously unwelcome by referers. A more effective approach for the hospital, described here by an administrator, is the control of demand by limiting the *promotion* of referrals:

> It was earlier this year when we were *trying* to review the type of patients that GPs were offering for treatment but we rather side-stepped that one because ... [the psychiatrist] wanted to wait; the last thing we wanted to do was to get a *flood* of referrals that we couldn't respond to.

Controlling demand by limiting the promotion of referrals is a feature, too, of the day hospital's relations with other consultant psychiatrists in the area psychiatric hospital. They are not actively encouraged to consider the day hospital for use with their in-patients on being discharged home.

In practice this caution is effective. Concern to avoid 'opening the floodgates' for referrals from other psychiatrists results in only about 8% of day hospital admissions coming from that source.

(2) ACTIVE DISCHARGE A second way of preventing any blockage is to discharge patients whenever possible. Given the widely recognized problems which characterize diagnosis and prognosis in the field of psychogeriatric medicine, it is clear that the discharge decision is a topic for considerable discretion (see, for example, Marsden 1978). Patients whose condition has deteriorated as well as those whose condition has improved may be discharged. This is not to imply that patients are discharged in a way that could be adjudged clinically premature. (Such a judgement is not a part of our evaluation of the hospital. We shall be returning to this point in Chapter 6.) Goldstein et al. (1968), in a study of a psychogeriatric day hospital, noted that despite a 42% discharge rate, in the first year of operation they could not claim that patient improvement had resulted in the discharge of even one case. Studies by Blake (1968) and McDonald et al. (1971) also show low rates of discharge due to patient improvement. Goldstein and Carlson (1976) have generally criticized day hospitals which operate discharge policies which are conservative.

Nevertheless the day hospital that we are studying has ceased treatment, at the end of a year, of about 70% of the patients admitted in that year. There are several ways in which this is achieved, and the range of discharge destinations for day hospital patients reflects the fact that clinical improvement is not the only criterion used. Cases of clinical improvement to the extent of eliminating the need for day care altogether actually account for only 12% of discharges, although a further 7% of patients are considered to have improved to a point where they have become acceptable to transfer to other forms of day care.

By far the largest group of discharges (51%) is due to deterioration in the patient's condition: 32% go on to a long-term bed in various parts of the hospital system, 7% are admitted to beds in the acute sector, 6% become housebound and unable to attend and 6% of patients die. A further substantial group of discharges (20%) occurs because patients and/or relatives refuse to continue attendance. The remaining 10% of discharges are accounted for by a variety of reasons which are not related to improvement in the patients' condition.

Although comparisons with other studies are difficult due to the different categorizations used, these figures do not seem untypical of statistics on psychogeriatric day hospitals presented elsewhere in the literature. From studies by Blake (1968), McDonald et al. (1971) and Goldstein et al. (1968), the average rate of discharge due to patient improvement is about 3%. The day hospital we are studying is thus achieving a higher than average rate in this respect, but this may be accounted for by variation in definition of what constitutes 'improvement'. As for those cases discharged but not accounted for in terms of improvement, Goldstein et al. (1968) are alone in using a 'self-discharge' category accounting for 20% of cases. This is the same level as 20% 'refusals' at the day hospital. Transfer to in-patient care is not a caregory utilized by Goldstein et al. (1968) but they do report 20% discharge rate due to 'deterioration'. Combining figures for 'deterioration' with discharge to in-patient care (on the assumption that such patients have also deteriorated) in the three studies, produces varied rates: Blake 13%, Goldstein 20%, McDonald 49%. This compares with 50% for the day hospital. The variation may be accounted for by differences in availability of in-patient accommodation and/or tendencies for the day hospitals to retain patients. The latter suggestion gains some support from the way in which the percentage of patients continuing to attend (Blake 67%, Goldstein 58%, McDonald 50%, the day hospital 33%) seems to have an inverse relationship to the percentage of discharges due to deterioration.

There are other studies which present a seemingly more optimistic picture of discharge patterns. For example, Morton et al. (1968) report that 52% of those admitted to a 'psycho-socio-geriatric assessment unit' were discharged directly back to the community, but of these fifty-two cases (N = 100), twenty-three in fact left for a 'welfare home'. Pitts (1974) reports that 71% of patients are discharged 'back to community' but this is used as a residual category, the only other specified categories being 'died' or 'discharged to other hospitals'. Thus here, as in other studies, it is clear that clinical improvement is only one reason for discharging patients.

A policy of active discharge achieves patient flow from a consultant's perspective. However, even when accompanied by intermittent readmission, it creates problems for others, particularly for social workers and relatives who still have the task of providing continued help to the patient at home. One relative explained what she saw as her difficulty:

> MRS Z: 'They thought of puttin' her down to this day centre for two days to take her out of the hoose, to stop thinking about herself, and she got on great ... Then they thought, well there was always somebody worse than herself, other folk waitin' to get in; she was stopped the Tuesday and see within a fortnight, she went back a wee bit, this was her only goin' one day and then oot the blue – two month after that they stopped the two days.'
> INTERVIEWER: 'What do you think is going to happen in the future with her?'
> MRS Z: 'Well a' I can see she's got to look forward to if they stop the day centre again she's jist goin' to go away again. It'll be a full time job just to try and keep her like – goin.'

(3) ALTERNATIVE SERVICES A third way for the consultant to achieve patient flow is for the hospital to serve as a gateway to other services. Some patients may pass along routes to other forms of day care, particularly to services provided by the local authority (as opposed to the National Health Service), that would not otherwise have been open to them.

The difficulty here is similar to the way in which GPs' use of the day hospital sometimes accentuates the problems of hospital staff. A referral from the day hospital to obtain some other form of service provision increases the effective demand for this service and denies it to a social-work client who might otherwise have used it (although in practice this route is not a busy one, with only 6% of patients being discharged from the day hospital to social work department facilities).

(4) USING BEDS The fourth approach to seeking turnover in the population of patients entails the day hospital, and particularly the consultant, making use of a small number of beds in Park Hospital in a variety of ways and in close association with the day hospital. 'Short-term beds' entails admission of a patient to Park Hospital for a strictly limited period. 'Shared beds' entails two patients alternating in their use of the bed by week or by days of the week. And 'emergency beds' are beds reserved exclusively for admitting patients taken suddenly ill while actually attending the day hospital. Although not always in conjunction with a day hospital, similar flexible use of hospital beds for planned intermittent admissions has been developed elsewhere in response to a shortage of in-patient beds (Erickson and Backus 1973; Robertson et al. 1977).

From the consultant's point of view, short-term beds have clear advantages – as he explained:

> When you take somebody in here [Park Hospital] for long-term care, although they're elderly that can still be very long-term – years – so if you take somebody into a bed for long-term care that often means that's a bed out of commission for a few years, whereas if you can arrange it for short-term admission you could pass perhaps fifteen or sixteen people a year through it, that's how I see it.

Such short-term admissions to Park Hospital are used extensively. Approximately 21% of patients attending the day hospital in any one year are offered this facility. It is a significant means of providing short-term in-patient care when compared with the very limited number of cases successfully referred for geriatric or social-work facilities.

Short-term beds may not however offer a solution to the problem as perceived by relatives.

> Mrs H: [The GP] told me there and then that there was a short-term bed and it would be available soon and when my mum was admitted I was to go to him and he would give me a certificate. I was to take a week ... anyway that's how she got in and it was just when she was due to come out that I went to see [the social worker] if there was not a possibility, because quite honestly the way I was feeling I was dreading having to try and cope all over again and I could only see the same thing happening. I had just got to the very end of the line and could take no more and please somebody help me. I was trying everywhere for help, there was no help available.' (Tearful)

Relatives may be reluctant to accept that they have not obtained a long-term bed. This reluctance creates difficulties for social workers and for ward staff, who have to deal with dissatisfied relatives. Furthermore, short-term admission require a redefinition of priorities in the allocation of beds. These may not be readily accepted by administrators who wish to ensure, on paper at least, that there is maximum utilization of beds.

From the consultant's point of view, using 'shared beds' has clear advantages. Although this practice is developing, the numbers involved remain very small and the innovation is less significant than the use of 'short-term beds'. However, on this, as on other points, the interests of different staff groups sometimes diverge. For example, the innovation initially met with resistance from a nursing officer on the grounds that the administration would be too complex. With shared-bed arrangements, too, the relatives may be receiving a service which is different from that which they had expected. Again social workers and ward staff may have to cope with the resentment which results. The problem with one case was described in an account by a ward sister at a hospital meeting, as recorded in our field notes:

> And some of the relatives were getting nasty but she had made it very clear that it wasn't her fault that the patient was in her present situation with only a shared bed. The social worker commented that they didn't have another bed for her. The ward sister continued and said that she had told the relatives to use the official complaints procedure if they weren't happy with the way the patient was being treated. The consultant said he thought the ward sister had dealt with this very well indeed. This was a situation which couldn't be helped. There was a problem in the other shared bed as well. There was no way in which they could do anything at present except note that the patient was needing extra help ... The social worker said ... that things at home were really bad. The girl had come to the relatives' group. She was very angry and frustrated and needed to have her complaint heard. The social worker thought she had got a lot out of the group and went away feeling much better ... The consultant said that in this case he didn't think the hospital had anything to hide. They could contact MPs and all the rest if they liked.

In such cases GPs, police and other community services, as well as social workers, have to cope with patients and relatives during the period in which patients are at home.

Also, as a part of the arrangements for co-ordinating day hospital places and ward beds, the consultant prefers to retain some vacancies at the day hospital for emergency use. We do not mean to imply that the consultant's manoeuvres are purely tactical. He also exercises very considerable power rooted in his professional and legal position as consultant-in-charge of the hospital. Nevertheless it is argued that only by preserving some flexibility and by tolerating the less than 100% occupancy rate that this entails, is it possible to make any attempt to cope with relatives' holidays, emergencies and the other unexpected demands on the system. Thus what may be seen by administrators as a hospital operating at less than its full potential is viewed by hospital staff as being one stretched to its limits.

Day hospital nursing staff

The second major constituent group of the day hospital is the nursing staff. This group includes the sister, a senior enrolled nurse, a community nurse, as well as nurses and auxiliaries. Amongst such staff there is, as amongst other groups, a general agreement that it is highly desirable to maintain a throughput of patients. Like the consultant, nursing staff have strategies for maintaining patient flow.

The first step involves negotiating with relatives about their understanding of the terms of the admission. The following extract from our field notes illustrates this point:

> The hospital is now beginning to be full up. This of course was a position which was anticipated but the crunch has now come and sister and the social worker were discussing what has to be done about it. Some patients have been coming to the hospital now for seven months or so ... Both the social workers and sister felt that there had to be some system initiated by which when patients were admitted to the hospital their relatives were clearly informed that there would be an assessment at such and such a point and the admission would only be for, say, three months. Relatives would be told that the patient would be discharged and might then be readmitted but they would then be prepared for the discharge in a way in which they are not at the moment. Of course both sister and the social worker agree that there will be some patients who cannot be discharged at the (say) three-month point, and it would have to be accepted that some cases would be an exception to this general principle; but the point is that relatives would be prepared for the discharge decision as a general rule.

Nursing staff also feel that patients should be very carefully selected to ensure that silt-up does not occur. Austin et al. (1976) and Pathy (1969) have noted the importance attached by day hospitals to selectivity in admissions policies. Also, Goldstein et al. (1968) state in their review of a day hospital that, 'Our ability to achieve goals and to utilize our resources in the most efficient and effective manner depends, to a large extent, on the proper selection of patients.' As one nurse explained in an interview:

> It's very easy to take the first ten people that come along, you have to be selective ... each person should be assessed, and if you can't do something therapeutically for them, there is no point in filling the place and then you can't admit somebody else who could benefit, and it's a hard thing to say, 'Well, I'm sorry, you're not suitable'. Everybody isn't suitable.

The problem as ever is that the pursuit of sectional interests creates trouble for other groups. Changes in control of admissions to one unit can have far-reaching consequences for the operation of an entire system of service (Silverman and Val 1975). Selectivity runs counter to the needs of GPs who want assistance in providing care for the patients who present them with the greatest difficulties. Selectivity can also be the focus of criticism and resentment from staff of long-term wards in Park Hospital, who feel that they are then left to cope with the residue of 'bad' cases. Some comments from ward staff illustrate this tension:

> Maybe I'm trying to put barriers up and all that, because other people have got a better job than I have [laughs]. We seem to get the heavy end of the stick, I mean it's heavy nursing right enough in our ward. Then you go over to [the day hospital] and see the lovely kind of surroundings and all that and the nice patients sitting there doing a bit of knitting and what have you, and come back to the ward again a wee bit down in the dumps, a wee bit demoralized. I think their grading is pretty high, that's how I say I think they're far too selective. I never see anyone that to my mind – as I can see there – is what I would say a real good going dementia.

However, since 77% of referrals to the day hospital subsequently become day patients, the staff of the day hospital do not appear to be operating a very rigorous selection policy. Many cases are not admitted because of the patients' circumstances, rather than because day hospital staff make a decision about suitability. A maximum of 10% of referrals are actually rejected by the day hospital staff as being unsuitable. Thus GPs are being relatively successful in advancing their criteria for admission suitability to the day hospital. However, with 32% of patients going on to long-term beds, the day hospital is doing little to divert patients from the ultimate destination of in-patient care (although it may be delaying their entry somewhat – a point that we shall take up in Chapter 6). This would not be entirely unusual. Greene and Timbury (1979) describe a geriatric psychiatry day hospital thus: 'The role of this day hospital has not therefore been to avoid admission or to expedite discharge or even greatly to postpone admission to long-term in-patient care.' The views of the ward staff are rooted in the very real difference which they perceive between the severity of conditions in the in-patient and day-patient populations, but it is by no means clear that the selection practices of the day hospital staff affect the standard of patients ultimately admitted to the wards.

For social workers the emphasis placed by the day hospital staff on maintaining patient flow increases the task of finding alternative provision for patients in order to prevent admission to the day hospital and to promote discharges. Relatives too may not always perceive the activities of nursing staff aimed at promoting discharges as being helpful. We shall return to this point when we deal specifically with relatives' interests.

In the face of the potential opposition which comes from reaction to the nursing staff's approach to patient flow, a range of organizational tactics has arisen. Sometimes, groups are able to use the power which they exercise by virtue of their professional prestige, bargaining position, organizational locale or control of resources. Sometimes, power is most effectively exercised by groups entering into alliances, the one with another. It is notable that the consultant psychiatrist is not amongst those whom we listed as being inconvenienced by nursing staff. Indeed the interests of consultant and staff are very close on this matter. For in practice the staff at the day hospital and the consultant often share the same problems with regard to turnover.

In attending hospital meetings we observed a number of tactics entailing collusion between consultant and day hospital staff designed to ensure continued patient movement. Some cases about which the consultant has reservations regarding suitability are accepted for 'a trial' or a 'period of assessment'. By doing this he recognizes the professional expertise of the nursing staff who are largely responsible for this 'assessment' and also holds open the possibility of review and discharge should admission prove to have been ill-advised. The consultant may agree to admit a case but hold open the possibility of the patient being discharged to other facilities in the future. The number of days per week which the patient is allocated can be limited. Any case setting a potential precedent is treated cautiously. Admission criteria are flexible and, although this does not often happen, on occasions cases which might otherwise be considered suitable may be refused admission if staff are anxious about imminent 'silt-up'. Another strategy adopted jointly by consultant and staff when places are under heavy demand is to delay the decisions on some patients and thus regulate the rate of admission. Finally there is a variety of tactics to reduce frequency of attendance and thus edge patients towards the door, – for example, in this extract from our field notes on a hospital meeting:

> Sister asked if she could reduce Mr I's attendance to once per week. The consultant agreed. It was also agreed that they should reduce Mrs Q's attendance to once per week, working towards her eventual discharge. The consultant said, 'Yes, of course, they must work towards discharge.'

The idea that patients should 'work towards' discharge is used by staff in their direct dealings with patients who are encouraged to accept the view that patients should themselves be anticipating discharge as a normal feature of the hospital's services. On occasions, too, the fact that the consultant can 'keep tabs' on a patient after discharge, review the case and readmit if necessary, eases decision-making with increased turnover in view.

General practitioners

The interests of GPs are amongst the most crucial to the operation of the day hospital, since the accepted admission pathway and the one followed by the vast majority of patients is via their GP to the consultant in charge. Only 12% of patients arrive in any other way. The GPs' interests in maintaining patient flow are primarily concerned with their problems in obtaining services for patients who are proving troublesome. As Shulman and Arie (1978) have shown, in their analysis of the reasons for the fall in admission rates of old people to psychiatric units, it is probably becoming more difficult for demented people to be admitted to psychiatric hospitals. For many GPs psychiatric cases represent a severe burden. Pressed by relatives, and their own concern for the patient, the GP's major task often becomes the search for some form of hospitalization. Carney et al. (1970) have described the burden imposed upon GPs by these patients in the form of calls and consultations. Williams (1980) has reported the variety of headings that GPs use to describe such patients in attempts to gain access to hospital facilities. From this point of view, the day hospital represents a new and welcome additional point of referral. As one GP explained: 'I think, speaking as a GP outside, I can see the benefits greater than I can from the inside. Before there was very little I could do for psychogeriatrics.' Jones and Munbodh (1982) report that 65% of GPs referring patients to one day hospital for the demented elderly described patients' attendance as reducing demand for GP care and treatment.

The pressure which GPs exert on the system is clearly demonstrated in the hospital meetings. Although no GP actually attends these meetings, other staff frequently quote GPs' letters and telephone calls, and refer to the fact that GPs are under pressure. The following examples are from our field notes:

> The GP in his letter had said that the patient was demented, but the consultant suggests that it is more a case of agitation. He read out an excerpt from the GP's letter in which the GP said that he was under strong pressure from the matron of the home to have her removed.

> She had originally been accepted as a patient at the day hospital not because staff thought they could help her but because she had great nuisance value over a long period of time at her local GP group practice.

Of course, the type of case for which hospital service is most welcome is that which the GP regards as the most severely ill, most unlikely to be able to remain at home with relatives, even with domicilary support, or most likely to present some 'crisis' through nocturnal wanderings or whatever. Yet as an administrator explained, it is precisely this type of referral which causes problems for patient flow at subsequent points in the system. Referral of one type of patient at one stage may 'silt up' the system at another:

> GPs had very fixed ideas about the *sort* of patients that were suitable for [the day hospital] and invariably a lot of these patients were, obviously, in the more advanced stages of mental deterioration and therefore the scope to help these patients was limited.

Certainly staff see GPs' referral practices to the day hospital as conflicting with their interests, and such conflicts as endemic to the system of psychiatric care. In one interview a nurse described this problem:

> [GPs] want the patient removed from the community and put into a ward, because that takes the onus off of them and they're safe and secure in a hospital ward, and you are always going to come up against the problem of that because you are going to try the opposite and reverse it and keep the patient in their own home and the GPs wouldn't like that.

These tensions reflect very real differences in the criteria which GPs and hospital staff apply when considering possible admission. The GPs' requirements are for facilities which will help them cope with any elderly patients who are making, in their opinion, excessive demands on their time and energy. It is this need which brings them into conflict with day hospital staff who feel that they must retain selectivity in order to avoid 'silting up' their part of the system. However, these conflicts do not always emerge explicitly. (In practice the vast majority of referrals are accepted.) As we are explaining throughout this chapter (as elsewhere in the research), each group is heavily dependent upon several other groups for the accomplishment of its day-to-day work. We have noted that there is widespread acknowledgement that this work should be conducted in accord with the overall aims of 'patient flow'. A group risks endangering co-operation with others and risks a challenge by others to its own image of success if it casts aspersion upon the intentions of other groups. So typically nurses describe GPs' activities as the result of failure in communication and understanding, and not as a direct challenge to the successful function of the hospital. As one senior nurse commented:

> The trouble really has been caused by GPs not really understanding what the unit's about and thinking that we can just accept people willy-nilly sort of thing ... We do have to discharge an individual after a period of time, something which I think the GPs still haven't quite got to grips with. I think they imagine that once they are in, and until there's a marked improvement, that the patient will remain with us, but this is not the case ... I would like to see us being able to – educate, shall we say, the GPs a bit better.

This is a very familiar tactic within organizations for diffusing ideological or interest group conflict and maintaining a sense of coherence in the system as a whole (see Thompson 1980).

Ward staff

We did not initially think of staff in Park Hospital, the larger institution in the grounds of which the day hospital has been built, as a constituent group of the day hospital. But links between the two hospitals developed in the pursuit of patient-flow objectives, and in several ways that we have already mentioned this group of staff are an intrinsic part of the operation of the day hospital. The two sets of buildings are very close. Park Hospital has psychogeriatric wards. Some senior nursing staff have responsibility for nurses in both hospitals. The consultant in charge of the day hospital places is also in charge of some beds in Park Hospital. From the perspective of the staff of Park Hospital, the day hospital is seen as a potential supplement to their resources and an aid to the discharge of long-term patients. As Wadsworth et al. (1972), Whitehead and Mankikar (1974) and Goldstein and Carlson (1976) report, many day hospitals for the elderly operate similarly in close conjunction with in-patient facilities.

The use of the day hospital as ward staff would wish conflicts with the aims of other groups. There is conflict with the day hospital staff. A strategy which would enhance patient flow out of in-patient wards would generate problems for the day hospital by blocking that part of the system if patients did not move on. An administrator explained:

> Initially they [in Park Hospital] wanted us to have patients in the ward over ... really what they were looking for was making us an extension of diversional

> therapy which would have been no good at all, just bringing the patients in here and [the day hospital] doing something ... but that would have snowballed if you know what I mean, we would have ended up as an extension of diversional therapy and that would have been all.

Similarly, for the consultant psychiatrist, admitting someone as an in-patient to the day hospital can only be advantageous if there is a definite prospect of discharge and freeing an in-patient bed. A nurse noted that without discharge the hospital is left with one patient effectively occupying two places,

> but we [in Park Hospital] still thought it could have been used in the event of there being places, y'know for example, there's not always twenty-five in every day and on the days when they weren't up to their full total possibly a few patients from the wards could go over but [the psychiatrist] didn't agree with this outlook at all. He has stated quite categorically that unless there is some hope of that person living outside the hospital, wherever, he doesn't see that they have a place in the day hospital.

In practice, the day hospital is not playing any major role as a stepping-stone for outward movement of patients from Park Hospital. For example, in one twelve-month period there was only one attempt, and that unsuccessful, to use the day hospital to discharge a long-term patient.

As the nurse that we quoted above implies, the consultant has made a policy decision about the role of day hospital places in discharges from Park Hospital. Although there is not often negotiation on this point, there are examples in hospital meetings of cases where Park Hospital staff press for the discharge of recent admissions whom they consider to be inappropriately placed. In the case described in the following field note, the patient had previously attended the day hospital but had been admitted to a bed in Park Hospital. The ward charge-nurse is now suggesting a trial period at home with a view to eventual discharge, with day hospital support:

> The nurse, however, stuck to her guns and returned again to the question of the patient. The nurse put it this way. 'I am sorry to keep pushing this patient, but he had made a request to go home and he is the best of the patients that we have on the ward' and so the nurse suggests that perhaps the meeting needed to reflect on what they might be able to do with the patient. However, the social worker feels it necessary to point out that ... the patient's wife would go along with any demands that were made upon her but would not in fact be able to fulfil the demand ... [because she will not be able] to accommodate her husband when he does return home. Thus, it would be more difficult to help the family and to accommodate the patient since there would have been a trial run of his going home which is what he seemed to want so much and that would fail and that would lead to all kinds of difficulties and strains for the family. At this point the consultant intervenes by almost thinking aloud, 'How would it be if – suppose that when he goes home his diabetes gets bad and he might flare up. We could give him a weekend at home and then persuade him to come back.' The social worker says this might be a problem because he won't want to come back, it is quite true, but on the other hand, she suggests perhaps the family won't be able to bear any more, so that we need to move rather tentatively, 'we need to see how things go'. The consultant then recapitulates from what has been said and attempts to draw some

> conclusions. He says, '*Although he is good in the hospital, the problem is in the home and the family where he might behave differently and this arena is the important one.*' The social worker says that she would like to speak to the family first, before she announces any plans in respect of the patient. The nurse again reiterates her apologies; she says, 'Sorry to go on about him, but he is the best patient in the ward'. [Italicized words underlined in original note.]

The outcome in this instance is ultimately determined by the fact that the consultant supported the social worker in resisting ward staff pressure to obtain a discharge from Park Hospital. We noted above that in spite of significantly different interests, groups are in various ways heavily dependent upon each other for co-operative activity. This would explain why the difficulties which a discharge might create for the social worker outweighed in the consultant's mind the arguments of ward staff in favour of discharging the patient. These were arguments which the consultant might otherwise have welcomed as 'facilitating patient flow'. In a contrasting case, Park Hospital staff were more successful in obtaining a discharge after the social worker was pressed into offering assistance of accommodation from the social work department. This move fulfilled the needs of the ward staff in moving out a patient they considered inappropriately placed and the the needs of the consultant by releasing a short-term bed for his further use, and avoided the threat of filling a day-hospital place permanently.

We have here very specific instances of the general point that we are making throughout this chapter. Much of what takes place in connection with the movement of patients around the system can be explained as the pursuit of parochial interests cast as organizational goals.

Social workers

The social worker, as a member of the team of day-hospital staff, is involved in making decisions about admissions and discharges to an extent which is not always evident in this type of setting (for comparison, see Wadsworth et al. 1972). She accepts the general principle of the need to maintain patient flow in the light of particular patient needs. However, for her more than for other staff this has to be tempered with concern for the needs of the family unit. For in practical terms it is the existence or not of a family capable of looking after the patient that largely determines the nature and possibility of discharge 'to the community'. Because such practical concerns are not uppermost in the minds of other staff who see themselves primarily as members of a hospital, a medically oriented view may be rather different. Peach and Pathy (1978), for example, have noted in the context of geriatric care that the traditional medical history and examination pays no significant attention to the social support a patient needs. A social worker made the point thus:

> Well a social worker offers a wider view of the patient. I think that's putting it in a nutshell. . . . First of all I think the medical team would see the social worker as a resource person, I think that is part of it but it is not all of it, in fact it's not anywhere near what the social worker can offer to the team. . . . They can be quite educative in widening the medical team's point of view. The medical side is usually very narrow, I don't mean they're narrow people, just that they see it as a medical

problem, bring them in, do a thing, cure, home or whatever to provide and that's it ... I thought that they had to understand what a social worker was, now that is not an easy thing to do without causing a lot of resentment.

Although differences in perspectives of medical and social-work staff reflect differences in training and professional attitudes, they reflect too the very different practical interests of different groups of staff. The one is primarily concerned with tasks *within* the boundaries of the day hospital, the other with tasks *without*. Relatives' support for discharged patients is a major part of the social worker's day-to-day work. So some resistance to discharge on the part of the social worker reflects her concern about limited family support, which largely accounts for the absence of any significant number of cases of successful discharge of long-term Park Hospital patients.

Naturally, such a pattern works against the interests of consultant and day hospital staff as well as the ward staff. Potentially therefore the social worker is in an isolated position, with interests quite distinctly different in key respects from all other staff groups. This potential isolation is accentuated by the fact that the interests of her own social work department are also distinctly different from those of the hospital system. But an isolated position is intolerable for any group within the hospital because, as we have noted, each is heavily dependent upon the co-operation of others. Thus the social worker must achieve a *modus operandi* in which the practical constraint of having to arrange relatives' support is modified by a co-operative approach towards achieving the goals of the most powerful of the day hospital's staff groups. The social worker must mediate between the interests of the hospital and those of the social work department. She explained this in interview:

When you're a social worker in this kind of setting it's sometimes difficult to define where you are, who is it I work for and who is my client. Is it the patient, is it the hospital, is it the relatives or is it the social-work department? Who am I trying to help? Sometimes when you have the traumas and the dramas of the job then you're stuck right in the middle, and you really have to try ... so I try very clearly to define in my own mind whether I am trying to please the ... I would never try to 'palm off', if you like, a psychogeriatric patient in a 'Part 4' accommodation, one, because I think that would be wrong, but two, I certainly think it would be wrong for the unit as a whole because if I say all sorts of things and I persuade them, as you can do at times, to take somebody who is totally inappropriately placed, that would please the consultant and that would please us here as well as at the unit but it will not please them [i.e. Part 4 staff] as time goes on and then I won't be believed the next time, so there are things like that that are very frustrating.

In practice the bargaining which ensues does not lead to substantial numbers of patients being discharged from the day hospital to social work department facilities. Only 6% of patients leave the day hospital in this way, and only a very small proportion of referrals dealt with by the day hospital is actively rerouted from Health Service to social work provision. However, a variety of short-term co-operative arrangements between the services has occurred and the negotiations giving rise to these are regularly reported in our field notes. For example, one patient, Mr A, was coming short-term from the care of his relatives to take up a hospital bed. In order to make a bed available, Mr B was being discharged from the hospital to local authority Part 4 accommodation for a similar short period but under the clear understanding that he would be readmitted to the hospital at the end of that period and that the current move did not represent a termination of any 'psychogeriatric' designation. On other occasions the bargaining involves the social worker having to run counter to the interests of the day hospital staff by persuading them that other facilities are also suffering from pressure of demand.

Relatives

Although relatives are never present at hospital meetings, their influence on decision-making is considerable. We have described their impact upon the work of the social worker. Relatives' interests also have an effect on the psychiatrist's decisions about the form of treatment to which patients should be allocated. Although we should be careful in treating relatives as a homogeneous group it is because we consider them to be a significant constituent party to the day hospital that we are concerned with their perception of and influence upon patient flow. Rathod and Vandrey (1971), for example, report that relatives' attitudes towards patients' disturbed behaviour is a major factor in the decision as to whether to admit the patient to in-patient or day care. Bergmann et al. (1978) report family support as the most important factor in retaining the patient in the community.

The extent of the intervention required by relatives varies according to the condition of the patient. Many relatives expect and often experience a progressive deterioration, and their interest is therefore in obtaining a service which will provide relief on a long-term basis. Ultimately, for many relatives, the need is for the patient to be admitted to a permanent hospital bed. This does not always coincide with the views of the medical service. For example, the efforts of relatives to acquire beds create problems for the GPs and other community-based services. In cases where relatives want a more extensive service than is being provided, hospital staff may have difficulties in coping with dissatisfied relatives. Whereas most staff have an interest in maintaining turnover in the system as a whole, relatives have vested interests in what they regard as the appropriate admission and discharge of their particular patient. What relatives consider to be 'appropriate' depends very much upon the situation in which they find themselves (and, as we shall later discuss in greater detail, upon the way in which they construe this situation as a 'problem').

We interviewed relatives of twenty-three patients who attended the day hospital. At the time of day-hospital admission, the relatives of five of these patients had already requested that their patient be admitted permanently to in-patient accommodation. For these relatives the day hospital service was clearly less than they wanted and was viewed as the best alternative in a situation where more intensive provision was unavailable. In a further five cases the relatives were, at the time of the patients' admission to the day hospital, already forecasting the need for in-patient admission in the very near future. These relatives were usually coping with fairly severely demented patients and saw admission to a long-term bed as inevitable and likely to be necessary in the very near future. The comments of the daughter of one patient are typical:

> MRS N: '... As I say a month ago, when he really got so bad that Sunday night, I really had my mind made up, well there is only one place he can end up in and that's a mental home. I mean I am quite aware of that, I know fine that's what it will come to, because I don't see the two days at the day centre will make any difference to him at all.'

and later in the interview:

> INTERVIEWER: 'What do you think would make it reach the point where you had to ask for him to be admitted somewhere. Do you know or is that something you find out when you get there?'
> MRS N: 'Oh aye, we'll just take things as they come. I certainly, I don't see it going on much longer like this because one of the two of us is going to crack up if it goes on much longer. We just cannae see an end to it.'

In a large number of cases (eleven) the relatives wanted either a long-term period of day-hospital attendance with probably in-patient admission as the eventual outcome or at least indefinite day-hospital attendance to help support the patient at home (although, in practice, changes in circumstances or the patient's condition often led to different outcomes). Some relatives pointed out that their GP had explained the day hospital admission as support for the relatives with the prospect of long-term deterioration in the patient's condition eventually leading to hospital admission:

> INTERVIEWER: 'What do you think is going to happen in the future?'
> MRS MCH: 'I don't know, if she gets any worse – the reason she is going to [the day hospital] is, Dr B telt me, that she'll get worse, that I'll no be able to cope because she is going to get worse and he says I will never be able to cope with her, that they have her name doon for a bed to go in all thegither and I wouldnae mind that because she likes it and it wouldnae be that she would be in her bed all day, she would be up and mixing with other folk. He said it would be about eighteen months afore it was actually they could take her in.'

In only two cases (of depressed patients) did the relative have any clear expectation, in line with the general staff view, that the patient would be discharged from the day hospital after a short period of successful treatment.

Many studies of client use of services stress the relatively powerless position of client groups (e.g. Blaxter 1976). In many respects the relatives of psychogeriatric patients are no exception. Nevertheless, relatives as well as staff employ a range of tactics in order to gain their goals, and this leads to conflict.

From the staff point of view much of the confict is seen as communication failure. As we have already mentioned, denial of conflict is not uncommon in organizations. The practical solution, as staff see it, then lies in a fuller explanation to relatives of the real nature of the situation. For example, relatives do not share the hospital's perspective on discharge. The process may appear insensitive or incomprehensible. Staff are aware of this. The following field note on a relatives' group illustrates the point:

> When the social worker explained that there was a system of six-weekly reviews, the relatives were very worried about the patient being returned home because they

couldn't cope with the problems. In spite of some glossing to the contrary on the part of the social worker and sister, it seemed generally assumed that the basic condition of the patient would not have changed and that therefore the problems to be coped with on the part of the relatives would be the same.

Discharges must therefore be handled carefully. Any violent reaction from relatives causes the social worker considerable difficulty. One such instance was described thus in our field notes on a hospital meeting:

Apparently there was a considerable problem about one patient being discharged where the relative was told only a day or two before about the discharge and the social worker then got a lot of flak from the relative who complained about the way that 'you sit up there making your decisions' and 'don't know what is really going on down here' [i.e. in the home].

So that staff's attempts to obtain agreement from relatives on the way in which they are handling a case are not always effective. Where this fails, staff may partially respond to relatives' demands by providing a service of a less extensive nature than the relatives really require. Short-term admissions are the most obvious example of this ploy. As one member of staff explained: 'I think that's the point of the exercise, to keep the relatives from actually wanting a bed, or we would be in trouble.' Staff are aware that this tactic frequently does not meet the needs of relatives.

Relatives also pursue their own ends and they, too, have several tactics which they employ.

(1) CONTROL OF INFORMATION Relatives do control access to much information about the patient and this they may seek to use for their own purposes. The following discussion taken from our field notes illustrates one strategy which relatives may use to gain admission for the patient:

One patient has become very aggressive. The consultant wondered whether relatives had been hiding the aggression on admission. Other staff often felt that relatives did do that. Relatives were under the impression that, as with admittance to a local authority home, if they portrayed the old relative as being troublesome then they would not be admitted. On interview they therefore sometimes went out of their way to present a good picture by saying 'but we are just the opposite'. It sometimes turned out that, in fact, the patient was rather more troublesome than the relatives had pretended.

However, since relatives are handicapped through an imperfect knowledge of the operation of the hospital, they cannot always tell what information is likely to influence decisions in what way.

(2) RELIANCE ON STAFF Some relatives are anxious to obtain a bed but are very conscious of their own impotence in influencing the allocation of resources. Sometimes they pin their hopes on day hospital staff acting on their behalf:

INTERVIEWER: '... You feel you need a bed for her, you have coped for quite a long time now, how do you feel that there just isn't one?'
MRS M: 'Well there's no much we can do about it, this is it ... they [other

relatives] are pushing me to get my mother in you know and there is nothing I can dae, it is no up tae me ... I really don't know what is going to happen. I'm just depending on like [the social worker] someone like that to help me out and sort of push for a bed that's all, you know when the time comes and I have to have one. But if there is nothing there is nothing.'

Relatives certainly do not underestimate the power of staff when it comes to obtaining resources for day hospital patients and, even in very difficult circumstances, are reluctant to prejudice their chances of obtaining a bed by discontinuing attendance and risking falling foul of staff. The husband of one patient explained:

INTERVIEWER: 'So after she had her two weeks in hospital what happened when she came home? Did she go back to the day hospital then?'
MR Y: 'Eh, yes, although I said she was unfit to go they decided different. Well rather than upset the cycle, you know, because you were always hoping she would be taken in permanently, rather than break with them which would be rather silly, I said, "Yes". It was like leading an old horse that knew it was going to the knackers trying to get her in the bus.'

(3) HARASSMENT OF STAFF Relatives also wield some power in their ability to constantly harass the consultant psychiatrist and other staff. One extreme example of the conflict between relatives' interest in obtaining facilities for the individual patient and those of the hospital staff in maintaining patient flow was illustrated when the consultant described the difficulties experienced in attempting to institute a system of short-term beds. From his point of view it was necessary to be aware of conflict and to take steps to protect his position:

In this sort of work you're always looking over your shoulder at some relative who's going to complain at a high level; well, that's all right, if you can show that you've done everything possible: but, for example, if I've got a female vacancy tomorrow and said, 'Let's leave that till we line up a short-term patient' and in the meantime a tragedy occurred and there was some sort of enquiry, then I feel that I would be very vulnerable.

The tactic of harassing staff is also illustrated in the following extract from an interview with the relative of a patient who had failed to obtain an in-patient bed:

MR K: '... as we werenae satisfied with the way things were going ... I contacted my father's doctor, I said is there no way you could push it and he said, "Unfortunately no, but do you know anyone with a bit of influence?", no and he says, "Now I cannae put words into your mooth. Do you know anyone who can either cut red tape or cause a bit of a stir?" he says, "because I agree with you. I have spoken to your mother and I am your father's doctor" he says, "she shouldnae be left in that hoose" ... Anyway I got in touch with the head one and that in my mother's surgery and he said, "Right, I'm going to get in touch with [father's doctor]", and he says, "the two of us will start a wee bit pressure at the local level on to [Park]." Again he said, "If you know somebody, try and get them to put a word in that way" ... With my father being in local politics and being a Party man we got in touch with [the MP].'

Relatives may also harass the consultant when, having obtained admission of a patient to a short-term bed, they decide that it is not in their interests to have the elderly person returned home. We recorded one such case in the following discussion:

> Sister reported that Mr X's wife had said that she had been advised not to have him back. ... Mrs X says that she had 'double hernia' (this was something that she repeated at the last relatives' group). She had also told sister that Mr X abused her and she was generally very upset. The consultant asked who it was that had 'advised her not to have him back'. Sister said this wasn't clear but she imagined it might be the GP, according to Mrs X. Consultant: 'Oh no! This would not be so ... it's amazing how people manipulate the situation' [perhaps for my benefit] ... The consultant then elaborated a little on the way in which he encountered patients and relatives who played off one professional against another. Sister, the consultant and nurse all agreed that, 'They take up the short-term beds but then the barriers come up' [i.e. relatives say at first that they want a short break but once they've got rid of the patients they don't want to take them back].

In spite of the range of tactics used by both relatives and staff, conflict between them is generally muted. Open disagreement occurs only occasionally. When relatives 'go too far' then consultant, social worker and nursing staff assume considerable solidarity in the face of a threat to their mutual authority and control. Again, a field note on a hospital meeting provides illustration:

> The consultant asked the social worker if she felt the problem at home was being exaggerated. The social worker said that the wife was under a great deal of strain and the patient would have been a candidate for a bed very soon. She went on to say though that the way this patient had to be admitted really sticks with her, that the relative managed to pressurize them so much ... The consultant then went on to outline what had happened in this case. The son had phoned and gone into a tirade after which he hung up. He was threatening to go to the Press about the patient not being admitted as an in-patient. The consultant felt that the health board might not accept the decision of not admitting the patient because of the redecoration. The nursing officer asked if the whole fuss that the son had created had been a major factor in deciding to admit the patient. The consultant admitted that this was the case along with the fact that they were in a weak position because they had in fact had vacancies. Discussion continued and the crux of the staff's concern about relatives exerting pressure in this way eventually emerged in comments by the social worker. This man could go on to tell others that this is how the bed had been acquired and this could lead to widening rumours ... The social worker commented that, 'we learn as we go along'. In this case they had acted but they could now look at how they could better deal with this in future. She felt they had to teach this man that you cannot behave in this way. The community nurse commented that 'this manipulation does go on'.

Conclusion

It is a central theme of this research that an evaluative study should include the analysis of data on different groups' perceptions of success and their efforts to achieve it. In this chapter we have pursued some aspects of this general point in relation to the particular matter of patient turnover in the hospital. We have taken the view that an attempt to disentangle the meanings and pursuit of 'turnover' is an intrinsic part of the evaluative exercise.

Our attempt to unravel these meanings and the operational strategies which are consistent with them has involved a good deal of detailed description, both of the perspectives of different groups and of the workings of the institution. This detail has, cumulatively, displayed characteristics of the day hospital which are of central importance to questions of an evaluative kind. The picture of the day hospital which emerges is one of a pluralistic and segmented institution. The meaning of 'successful patient flow' for each party is heavily contextually determined, and the parties' success in expressing that meaning in practice varies with the degree of opposition that they meet when encountering the gambits of those who construe and pursue the hospital's successes in other ways.

Thus, for instance, GPs have few referrals refused, but their referrals are not encouraged as much as they might. Consultants have an additional resource but have experienced no significant easing in the shortage of in-patient beds. Day hospital staff have ensured, largely through influencing discharge rather than controlling admission, that patients go as well as come, but ward staff have largely failed to improve the in-patient discharge rates through day hospital auspices. The position of the social worker has minimized conflicts which might have arisen between the different health and social work perspectives, yet few patients flow freely between the facilities of health and social work. Relatives wield considerable potential power yet seldom exercise it as effectively as they might. These are examples of the kind of observations that we had made throughout the chapter in our attempt to link patient flow, as perceived by our respondents, to the performance of the hospital as a service institution.

Throughout, we have used the framework of a pluralistic approach to evaluation, which we set out in Chapter 1, to structure our data. In the next chapter we continue this approach as we describe how 'clinical cure' is variously used as a second criterion in the pursuit of success.

CHAPTER SIX

Success as Clinical Cure

Introduction

The so-called 'treatment model' of professional practice is often held up as the ideal which social workers, educators, criminologists and others concerned with demonstrating effective practice would dearly like to follow. The problem and its symptoms are clearly identified, a prognosis is established, a treatment is specified and administered, the effects are monitored and, in due course, the patient, client, pupil, offender (or whatever) is discharged, graduated or released 'cured'. The approach is the clinical equivalent of the model of rational planning which we discussed in Chapter 1. Of course medical practitioners themselves frequently point out that medical practice often only approximates to the medical model and is considerably less 'scientific' in that sense than lay observers are wont to believe. Nevertheless, both medical practitioners and laymen find it hard to conceive of a hospital that does not aim to 'cure' its patients.

As we explained in Chapter 4, the day hospital's ability to effect such a 'cure' is one of the main criterion advanced for assessing its success. In the field of psychogeriatric care, however, there are difficulties to a precise implementation of the 'treatment model'. Definitions of patients' problems in the field of psychogeriatrics are particularly imprecise (see Marsden 1978). Many of the categories are used to include a substantial range of clinical symptoms. Where a condition has been precisely described, often medical science has yet to discover a significant 'cure'. Many of the problems suffered by the elderly mentally infirm are of a multiple nature (Caird and Judge 1979), a difficulty which is compounded by the fact that many of these problems are social rather than psychiatric or medical in origin. Finally, psychogeriatrics is itself a very new branch of medicine (Kanowski 1978) which has as yet had little time to develop a specialized knowledge base when compared with the more established branches of the profession.

In the light of these difficulties we begin this chapter by describing how patients' problems are defined in the day hospital. Next we describe the range of facilities provided for patients in pursuit of an active therapeutic approach to their problems. We then assess the effectiveness of these measures on the basis of evidence available within the hospital. To anticipate our conclusion, we shall argue that the data leave considerable doubt about the degree to which hospital practices are consistent with the pursuit of success as clinical cure. Nevertheless the fact that the hospital is successful in these terms is widely reported within the institution. Towards the end of the chapter we shall therefore describe how this image of success is sustained.

The hospital's definition of the problem

A central feature of any organization operating in line with the treatment model of professional practice must be a relatively clear view of the nature of the problem that it is seeking to solve. In this section of the chapter we describe the way in which problem categories are assigned to patients entering the day hospital. Since ambiguity surrounds many of the diagnoses within geriatric psychiatry, it is these practical definitions of patients' problems that serve as the basis for treatment.

As we explained in Chapter 3, we collected data from a variety of sources. An important source of information in this chapter is the hospital records. Our data on the Tuesday meetings also reveal the way in which a definition of patients' problems emerges (or not) from group discussion.

The 'problem' in the records

We have already pointed to the way in which records are dispersed throughout the hospital and have explained that the several professions generate their own documents. A first complication in evaluating treatment is that a plurality of perspectives is reflected in the content of the files and, in particular, in the way in which patients' problems are defined.

The following examples are taken from cases in our six-month sample.

Mr M was assessed by several different professionals. The GP referral letter described him as follows:

> His main problem is that over the past few months he is becoming increasingly confused. The confusion is very variable and at times he is extremely lucid, however he does claim to see people wandering around his house and sitting outside waiting for him and has caused quite a few problems with his neighbours.

The nursing report defines the 'immediate problems' as 'auditory and visual hallucinations' and the first entry reads: 'Very pleasant man. Ambulant, continent, with indwelling catheter with which he copes very well. Slight confusion but communicates freely and socializes well.' The community nurse made a social assessment, reporting:

> He had gross memory impairment and suffered visual and auditory hallucinations, i.e. thinking people are coming into his room and sleeping in his bed. He lived

> alone but was supported by the lady who lived nearby (friend of his deceased wife) and he kept phoning her in the middle of the night complaining of the people who were in his house.

The psychiatric background report comments:

> There were distinct signs of memory impairment although, strangely enough, his memory for recent events seemed better than his memory for past events ... Mr M still seems able to appreciate being in his own home and I think perhaps admission to hospital would be premature at the moment.

A further example is the case of Mrs E. The psychiatric background report says:

> She often speaks about people trying to get into the house even though there is no one there and she accuses the others in the house of taking her money. On one occasion she spoke of being photographed while in her bath. It seems that she spends most of her time in bed except on the day she collects her pension. I think Mrs E's memory may be affected but the most prominent feature was the paranoid element.

The nursing report reads: 'Immediate problems; right arm support.' An early entry adds:

> Attended today. Very pleasant lady. Extensive bruising on left forearm due to fall. Support being worn. Personal hygiene requires observation. Unable to dress herself appropriately. Wearing two dresses. Social circumstances at home appear poor.

The home assessment by the community nurse says:

> She is a widow with gross memory impairment and confusion. She is basically continent but she doesn't clean herself properly after toileting. She is a very poor walker. Her appetite is good but even with impaired walking she still wanders. She was suffering from auditory and visual hallucinations and was imagining that everything she touched turned to gold.

The clinical examination adds as a 'diagnosis': 'Arteriosclerotic dementia.'

To add to this complication of a plurality of problem definitions in the records, background reports often indicate that it is not so much the diagnosis itself which is crucial in decision-making as the pressure that is being placed upon the hospital by some third party. Most often this is a relative or the patient's GP but is sometimes a neighbour or the care staff of a residential institution. For example the consultant psychiatrist reported on Mrs G:

> She has also been disturbing her son and her GP in the small hours. Some degree of this problem has been going on for years and she had a short spell in hospital to give her family some relief ... being in sheltered housing has not helped – may have made things worse by the nuisance to other residents.

The social background report on Mrs G explains a similar kind of problem:

> She is now quite disoriented in time and place and is unable to wash herself. She requires help with dressing because she dresses inappropriately, can no longer cook for herself. She is also doubly incontinent and very often defecates in the corridor of the unit. This of course is causing great distress to residents in the sheltered unit.

The summary assessment adds: 'I would therefore recommend that we attempt to alleviate the sheltered unit's burden and hopefully find something that will enable Miss G to continue in her own home.' The nursing report describes the immediate problem as: 'doubly incontinent. Upsets residents by defecating on the carpet in corridors.' And the psychiatric report adds:

> It seems Miss G has become gradually more forgetful, *but the real problem* is that she now tends to wander into the corridors and to be incontinent of faeces there. This is understandably distressing to other residents. [Italics ours.]

The conclusion we draw from these and similar data is that frequently no very precise and widely accepted definition of patients' problems serves as a starting-point for their clinical career through the hospital. To judge from the material in the hospital records there appear to be several reasons for this. First, patients are assessed by a variety of professions and the different professional groups appear to use different frames of reference in their diagnoses and assessments. Secondly, each profession tends to vary its assessment of each case over the period of referral and admission to the hospital. For instance the social worker may stress the confused state of a patient at one time while concentrating upon the consequences of this confusion for the staff of a residential institution at another time. Although these definitions are not always mutually exclusive they carry different emphases for courses of action to alleviate the problem. Thirdly, expressions of the problem move between expert terminology and lay accounts in somewhat commonsense terms. Again these expressions are by no means mutually exclusive but they tend to imply, on the one hand, that a solution lies in commonsense handling of the problem while, on the other, that the solution is a matter of considerable specialist expertise. Finally, the diagnoses vary considerably in their length from the short, 'arteriosclerotic dementia' of the medical examination to some accounts of the problem in psychiatric and social background reports which extend to a paragraph or more. Frequently such extended accounts contain several and sometimes different implications for action.

Moreover, as the files themselves indicate, a record of the problem is often less important than a record of the GP's or some other referral agent's pressure to offer a place.

The 'problem' in the meetings

Accounts of the patients' problems are a feature of the regular Tuesday meetings at which the majority of admissions are discussed. Here again a range of professional staff contribute to the process of defining the patients' needs. It is a particular feature of such accounts that they emerge as somewhat lengthy interchanges between staff.

The following is an extract from one Tuesday meeting at which a decision was made to admit three patients. Mrs N was admitted to the day hospital for a trial period as a case of dementia and because the relatives were needing help in caring for her. Mr and Mrs McE were admitted to the hospital for a period of assessment in part as a result of the demands that they were both making upon their local doctors. This is the extract:

CONSULTANT: 'I have been phoning in these referrals really knowing of your petrol position, thinking it would be a pity for you to come to [nearby town] one day maybe if there was another case there the next day, so I am trying to phone them in as they come up – eh – Mrs N was I think a pretty straightforward case of severe dementia looked after by her husband and the two daughters-in-law who seemed to have shared things. One of the daughters-in-law has been ill herself and more has fallen on the one I spoke to, Mrs N, they seemed to have worked hard and they are now looking for some help.'
SOCIAL WORKER: 'You saw one daughter and I saw the other one.'
CONSULTANT: 'Was that it, it is a daughter-in-law?'
SOCIAL WORKER: 'Oh you saw a daughter-in-law, I saw a daughter that was the lady who was in [another psychiatric hospital].'
CONSULTANT: 'Is that Mrs I?'
SOCIAL WORKER: 'She herself has been . . .'
CONSULTANT: 'Wait a minute now . . .'
SOCIAL WORKER: 'She said she was just recovering from a nervous breakdown, which had lasted two years really, and she is now just coming out of that and Mrs N herself, as you say, is very obviously demented.'
CONSULTANT: 'Very far gone.'
SOCIAL WORKER: 'Her husband is her second husband and they have been married well ten years since 1970 and the family that help him are certainly Mrs N's, his own family don't help very much at all. He is a very gentle sort of accepting man, he accepts what's going on. Now one of the things that has happened since you saw them was, and it hadn't happened before, was on Sunday. He was in the kitchen and he came through, he had shut the door where she was and he came through and the cushion of the settee had been put in front of the fire. It was alight but she had shifted it and had put it on to the settee again, she had . . . actually she must have put it in front of the electric fire, it caught fire and she must have shifted it and put it back on to the settee so that when he came in, there she was sitting with smoke belching out of this cushion and that obviously has worried him a great deal. There are a lot of dangers in that house because they live upstairs, very steep stairs, and he manages to contain her from getting near the stairs, but I think that is by the way he really works at it closing doors and what not. There is also a door which he has locked out onto the balcony which you know he is terrified she will fall over. She is obviously a very pleasant old lady and she has been a very good women I think.'
CONSULTANT: 'They're all Plymouth Brethren.'
SOCIAL WORKER: 'Yes.'
CONSULTANT: 'The whole family.'
SOCIAL WORKER: 'And this is very important to them, in fact one of the big things they do for him is that they always see he gets to the church on Sunday and to the meetings. There is a meeting on a Tuesday so that is all sort of catered for, it is most important. Then there was a funny kind of thing happened in a way, I was talking about day care and this daughter very quickly said, "No, no, that would not do, she isn't fit enough."'
CONSULTANT: 'I don't think I even mentioned [the day hospital] to them. I left it a very open thing but I put her on the waiting list, I think I simply said we would see if we could give them some support.'
SOCIAL WORKER: 'She was saying this that she couldn't get up and down the stairs now. She is – certainly she shuffles and I'm quite sure she could get up and down stairs.'
CONSULTANT: 'Yes, she has got out once or twice.'
SOCIAL WORKER: 'But they were being to me a little bit over-protective and

again it was a bed ... so again I said, "You know you are talking about an impossibility, certainly at the moment, and it is just not on, there isn't a bed" and oh that wasn't so good and the old man had sat very quietly listening to all this and I think that he got the idea that perhaps he wasn't going to get anything at all and it seemed to me that he took a little bit of courage in his hand to say, but I think day care might be a good idea because I think although they recognized that he is wonderful and does a great deal for this old lady I think perhaps they don't quite recognize what he's feeling and how much worry and strain it is for him.'

CONSULTANT: 'He had to nurse his first wife.'

SOCIAL WORKER: 'Yes, he is accepting it but I think he is, really he is very afraid for her, and of course this fire thing really frightened him a great deal that I would certainly say day care would be ...'

CONSULTANT: 'O.K. A trial anyway. Now Mrs D.'

SOCIAL WORKER: 'I was to look up my ... what I call my old referrals and I just forgot to do that doctor.'

CONSULTANT: 'But maybe I can [few words inaudible] just so that I can get the letter off. I know we decided not to do anything because she really wasn't bad at all. Now the other thing is, I saw Mr and Mrs McE, [nearby town].'

SOCIAL WORKER: 'Was she up?'

CONSULTANT: 'Yes [pause]. They seem to make great demands on the doctors. When I saw them they weren't distressed, they seemed quite happy and I think it was Mr McE whose memory is more affected than his wife, normally I would see two people separately but I couldn't in this case where two frail old people are sitting, so I had to do a kind of double interview. Mrs McE is fairly deaf but she was more in touch than her husband, he was at sea all his life, she was a teacher, they got married very late on, really the house was untidy but wasn't in a terrible state. The big problem seems to me what they do to the practice, and I phoned up to speak to Dr C to see why, so I spoke to the receptionist who at once recognized me [laughter].'

SOCIAL WORKER: 'That was actually the couple that when I went to see the doctors at the practice that was the one they said immediately, "Do you take couples?" and immediately the doctor said, "Well, this is a couple." And I went, like, to see the home-help organizer about them because they know all the things that go on really from day to day, and one of the things was that Mrs McE had had shingles and she still complains about this pain and she said to me whenever I went in, "Hello, how are you?" "Oh! you know," she was letting me see the pain she had, then she would go on and apparently she is in the habit of going out into the street and shouting for help, saying her husband is attacking her, and this is probably when he has had a drink, but when she was talking to me, when I saw them they were both in bed and the house is tidy outwith that bedroom, that bedroom is a total shambles.'

CONSULTANT: 'The sitting-room was a bit of a shambles when I ...'

SOCIAL WORKER: 'Was it? It was quite tidy but I think perhaps the home help had mebbe done ...'

CONSULTANT: 'Maybe there was somebody in, a neighbour was just leaving as I arrived.'

SOCIAL WORKER: 'Well certainly the home help had said the house is in a bad state so they obviously have a lot of problems with that. There is a daughter who lives in [nearby town] and who comes down and washes her mother but I think to get father washed is a different matter altogether, he doesn't really wash much at all. I didn't get a lot out of Mr McE because he was under the bed covers all the time.'

CONSULTANT: 'He was quite alert when I was there and memory affected but ...'

Social worker: 'The old lady, I don't know the word, is almost effervescent, gabbling on ...'
Consultant: 'She kept telling me about what a good man he was, its always a very ...'
Community nurse: [brief inaudible comment amongst laughter]
Social worker: 'Yes, she told me that – hm –'
Consultant: 'Maybe she thought I was planning to take him away.'
Social worker: 'She also said to me she had lived ... her father was an architect and they lived in this big house and he really was a fine fine man. She kept on saying this about all sorts of people. "Now there was this professor, who was an uncle of mine who was a fine fine man" but none of his family liked him y'know but she did, and that her father had ... she had another sister who she didn't like and when she got to about sixteen or so she left the home and of course she married, which was a big mistake because he was 'a brute' and that he drank, he was "an alcoholic of course" and that she had, then she sort of rhymed it off, "I had a daughter and she died and then I had a son and he died of cancer," then she married this man who was a gem and he is, it is funny because he was lying under these covers going [making funny noises]' [laughter]
Community nurse: 'A load of rubbish.'
Social worker: 'I said "Is he blethering?" or something like that and he said – Mmm, so obviously he was listening, saying "Here she goes again". But she wouldn't hear too well because of her deafness.'
Consultant: 'That's interesting because I have a picture of these two people very much at ease in each other's company. In fact I had to write out the questions for him because [laughter] she was so deaf and it was almost a sort of three-way sort of thing because he could hear me, but he couldn't remember [laughter] she couldn't hear me but she could. It was peculiar. Anyway do you think we can contribute anything here?'
Social worker: 'Well I think it would certainly help the community if we were taking them out. The thing about [a nearby town] is that it is a very good area for the follow-up things, that if we can get them for a period then I think day care – I think it is a good area for that kind of follow-up so I think to get them out of the house and to get something done I think perhaps it would help.'
Consultant: '... a difficult place to get to.'
Social worker: 'Yes.'
Consultant: '... so we would have to take them both on really for a period of assessment.'
Sister: '... for assessment, uhu.'
Consultant: 'Now for the next one is Mrs M ...

This extract shows how difficult it is to explain the admission process simply in terms of the clear diagnosis and prognosis that a treatment model would lead us to expect. It is also an apparent complication of these cases that they were admitted for a period of assessment or trial and no definite statement of the problem to be tackled appears to be made in the meeting. However, that is not at all an unusual procedure. As we have already observed in our discussion of patient flow (in Chapter 5), much decision-making in this day hospital consists of postponing decisions by recommending an assessment period. The treatment model leads us to expect some later point at which this assessment is clarified. In practice at the day hospital such clarification seldom occurs. The periods of 'assessment' and 'treatment' are frequently blurred with discharge, which takes place without a clear diagnosis ever having been made. All of this is far from the neatness and clarity of the rational decision-making model which the notions of 'cure' and 'clinical treatment' tend to imply.

Finally, in our attempt to give a picture of the way in which patients' problems are viewed within the hospital, we should mention that professional perceptions are significantly different from those which relatives hold about their patients. We deal fully in Chapter 9 with the topic of relatives' perceptions of the nature of the patients' problems but one point is relevant at this stage in our discussion. Although a strong treatment ideology pervades the responses of many staff, relatives of patients do not assess the performance of the hospital in such terms. They do not assign overall importance to the way in which they expect the hospital to improve the clinical condition of their patients nor do they advance a very precise clinical diagnosis of the nature of the patient's problems. Rather, as we shall later show at much greater length, the patient's condition for a majority of relatives is characterized primarily by a set of symptoms which are proving troublesome for them. For relatives the criterion of success is not so much the degree to which the hospital cures the patients of a diagnosed problem, as the extent to which the practical problems of caring for the patients are reduced.

An active therapeutic regime

We have explained that staff view the hospital as in institution which should be effective in the cure of its patients. This general point is given more concrete expression in the following account of the hospital services by a consultant psychogeriatrician:

> We can certainly in the day hospital look at the question of drugs, can't we? And although you cannot really improve somebody's memory, you can often do quite a lot to control things like agitation, which can be the thing that determines whether relatives want a patient in or not. If it's a depressed patient there again we're looking at the drug treatment and if its a paranoid patient we're looking at drug treatment. Of course they can't offer that in a social centre. We can offer occupational therapy in the sense of assessment and training as opposed to diversional. Then physiotherapy – now you don't need a day hospital to arrange physiotherapy but it's often more convenient to do so and, as you know, the physiotherapist attends the weekly meeting and incidentally provides some kind of link with the physiotherapy services outside. Diet – there's a number of our patients who I think have developed confusional states or at least where the confusion is added to the dementia if you like, through inadequate diet and we can, when we have a dietitian, make some kind of assessment of what the patient's diet really is and then try to correct any deficiencies one way or another. Chiropodist – of course we've got – and there again we have quite a few problems with feet. Again these can be dealt with outside the day hospital but sometimes it's more convenient to do so in this setting. Then outside I think that there are a certain number of cases where it just would not be practical to do anything ... so we've got a medical aspect to it. Physiotherapy, occupational therapy, chiropody, diet, nursing care of course, in a general sort of way, that can help too. So these are all things we can offer which a day centre can't.

In this section we take a number of these services and describe the facilities which are on offer within the hospital as components of the therapeutic approach towards patients' problems.

Psychiatry

The consultant psychiatrist is in overall charge of the psychiatric services of the hospital. He is most involved with patients at assessment for admission. For the majority of referrals he carries out, most often at the GP's request, an assessment based upon a domiciliary visit. In other cases his assessment is based on seeing the patient at the day hospital. A very few cases referred by other psychiatrists may be admitted without an assessment from the psychiatrist in charge.

The psychiatrist in charge chairs the discussion of cases at Tuesday meetings and is ultimately responsible for the admission decisions. This meeting takes up a major part of the one session which the consultant is allowed for his hospital duties. Once admitted, there is no routine contract between the psychiatrist and patients. Contact does occur from time to time, at the request of other staff who are in more regular contact with patients. These meetings between patients and the psychiatrist are usually brief. For the most part psychiatric treatment is confined to drug therapy. Once patients are admitted the psychiatrist bases most of his judgement about them upon the information which he collects from the sister in charge and from patient records of various kinds.

Staff see the psychiatrist's contact with patients (and, indeed, with staff) as rather limited. The following is one example of this feeling taken from an interview with a senior nurse:

> INTERVIEWER: 'How would you like to see the day hospital developing in the future?'
> NURSE: 'I would like to see more time from the psychiatrist. I would like to see at least another session from [the consultant] so that he could be doing on-going interviews and assessments on the psychiatric side of the patients and certainly that is an important thing, I think, that should be improved on . . .'
> INTERVIEWER: 'Yes, for what particular purpose?'
> NURSE: 'Well . . . to assess their psychiatric state from when he last saw them on a domiciliary visit and I think it would be very beneficial if he saw the patients before discharge . . . I think there should certainly be more group therapy going on. I would like to see a lot more group therapy going on.'
> INTERVIEWER: 'And do you see that [group therapy] as something which should be conducted by a psychiatrist? Or at least maybe yourself, somebody psychiatrically trained?'
> NURSE: 'Oh yes! I think it has to be somebody psychiatric trained, if you're going to do group therapy on them, if you're going to have groups and you're going to do therapy on them, and I think again that's something the consultant should be involved in as well, or a deputy of his, you know . . .'

Nursing

Patients' most extensive contact through their stay in the hospital is with nursing staff. As we have explained, a proportion of the nurses are auxiliaries who are not trained. These staff can offer, at best, sympathetic care and attention but only within a commonsense approach to the problems of the elderly mentally infirm. Throughout the day nurses carry out the routine procedures involved in dressing patients' wounds, bathing patients, administering medication, toileting (particularly the incontinent) patients, supervising meals and assisting the occupational therapist and diversional therapist with a range of social and diversional activities. Nurses also accompany patients who are going to Park Hospital for chiropody and other services and assist with hairdressing and shaving. Auxiliary nurses accompany the bus which transports patients to and from the hospital.

It is mainly nurses who complete the continuous set of records about patients within the hospital. They assumble a good deal of material including the nursing notes which form the basis of much decision-taking at the Tuesday meetings. The nursing-care plan is also particularly important. This is described by one nurse as follows:

> There is a care plan drawn up for every patient and I try to identify any potential problems that the patient is going to have, the confusion usually if it is specifically a senile dementia, disorientation, incontinence if there's any problems of that, vision, speech, if the patient's had a stroke and their speech is affected, if they're dysphasic, any problems at all that we can see is going to be a problem, aggressiveness, agitation, anything at all. That is put down in a column as a problem. We have then, we devise a specific aim, what do we want to do with that problem, do we want to try and orient them to their surroundings for the confusion, or incontinence, what regime do we want to use to try and retrain the bladder and the bowel; agitation, what do we do for that, you know, try and ... the aim is put down and then the actual way that we're going to deal with it, I write that down as well, you know how I want to deal with, and then each nurse, the nurses are all involved in a care plan, the nurses just go and take the care plan and they study that and they work along that line to the patient and every month, at the end of every month I review each care plan and see if we're doing anything with that problem, or if the problem has been eliminated, if the regime that we've drawn up to deal with the problem isn't working, is there anything else I can try so that ... you know, its done in pencil and we rub it out and try another plan. That'll try and alleviate the problem. That is for every patient there is a care plan drawn up and that is with specific aims of what we want to do for each patient in the department.

In practice such a rational and systematic approach is not clearly reflected in the decisions taken at the Tuesday meetings. As we have already explained, decisions at these meetings involve many criteria. Evidence on the systematic progress of patients in relation to very particular goals is not as clear-cut as this approach to a nursing plan would imply.

Nurses also complete Crichton scaling for patients. One nurse said:

> We use the Crichton scale for assessing the patient. It's a sheet and it gives you a score point. It's done up in points and the patient's mood is one of the aspects, dressing, feeding, incontinence, walking ability, you know, their mobility. There's eleven points on it and it goes from a score of one to five on each point and each patient that comes in here, we should really not accept anyone who has a Crichton scaling rate of over twenty-nine, because over twenty-nine means that a patient should actually be in a hospital bed and what we do is we mark this every week and each item is marked, as I say it goes from one to five, five is really very bad, and the patient's first rating might be, say thirty-four, and then with the on-going

> care plan, we do it every week and if the care plan is working out that scaling rate should come down.

Nurses explained to us that the hospital seeks to achieve a total score of eleven. Patients are then ready for discharge.

In our six-month sample of forty-five cases only twenty have Crichton scale ratings completed. This may be because in practice a Crichton scale is not completed regularly for all patients but may also be because these records are not always retained in the medical files. Of the twenty completed six are untotalled and thus, we presume, were not used as evidence in making a decision about subsequent patient career. However, it is clear from our sample that in most cases there is little variation in rating over the period of the patients' attendance.

The remaining fourteen cases show the following. (The periods over which the patients were rated ranged from one to sixteen weeks.) Five cases increased their rating evidencing deterioration. Seven cases lowered their rating evidencing improvement and two cases remained the same. In only three of the fourteen cases did the variation exceed three points. We could detect no clear relationship between the scaling and eventual discharge decision. For example, one case improved by six points over a four-week period, descended to a scaling of eleven and was discharged home, while another rose 9.5 points over twelve weeks to a final score of 30.5 and was also discharged home.

With the theme of this chapter in mind, we conclude that insofar as the Crichton rating scale is an accurate measure of the patient's clinical condition, then the majority of patients show very little improvement during their stay in the hospital. Alternatively we might conclude that the Crichton scale is unreliable. There is a good deal of evidence to suggest that decisions within the hospital do not take these ratings very seriously. Our preferred conclusion, in the light of the way in which these records are assembled and used within the hospital, is that they provide little support for claims about the clinical effectiveness of the hospital services.

General medicine

The medical officer is a local GP who attends the day hospital on a sessional basis for two afternoons each week. He is limited as a member of the decision-making team since he does not attend Tuesday meetings, although he does complete a set of records which contain both medical and psychiatric diagnoses. In addition to the two sessions each week, the medical officer is available at other times if requested by nursing staff since patients do not necessarily attend the hospital on the days on which the medical officer is present. The fact that the medical officer also attends Park Hospital for several sessions each week makes visits to the day hospital at a variety of times somewhat easier.

All new cases are seen by the medical officer within about one week of admission for a routine medical examination. This examination, the medical officer explained, is probably more thorough than that which most patients routinely receive from their own GP. However the treatment which patients subsequently receive from the medical officer is very similar to that provided in general practice. Indeed on some occasions the medical officer simply makes a formal referral back to the patient's GP. Few patients are treated continuously by the medical officer during their period of attendance at the hospital. Treatment which is given most often takes the form of drug prescription or minor medical procedures. Unless prescriptions are administered only at the day hospital the prescription is arranged through the GP to avoid the cost falling on the hospital budget. On a small number of occasions the medical officer refers the patient for further tests of a specialized kind. The medical officer does not routinely see patients prior to discharge.

Our overall conclusion is that the general medical service does not provide a unique treatment within the day hospital. However, it does compensate for some inadequacies in GP services and, in so doing, may well treat problems which might otherwise have remained undetected.

Occupational therapy

The day hospital has a full-time occupational therapist assisted by a part time diversional therapist. Other staff regard occupational therapy as extremely important within the hospital and all patients are automatically referred for occupational therapy at admission.

Shortly after each admission the occupational therapist completes a general 'activities of daily living' assessment. This assessment involves mobility, dressing, toileting, bathing and ability in the kitchen. The bedroom and kitchen in the hospital have been equipped to resemble those in a modern home. Some patients are given 'practice' in tasks that they find difficult. Some may receive as much as daily practice in dressing, or weekly practice in the kitchen. Generally, around six patients each week are receiving this kind of intensive service from the occupational therapist.

The occupational therapist also runs several reality orientation sessions and relaxation groups each week. The day room for the hospital has the usual reality orientation aids such as a notice-board containing some current affairs items, a date calendar and a sign displaying the day of the week. Sometimes too there are notices about the weather and season of the year. The occupational therapist takes the view, shared with the nursing staff, that reality orientation should not be confined to group sessions but should form a part of the overall day-to-day regime. Generally the hospital places rather less emphasis on systematic and intensive reality orientation than is to be found amongst the more committed advocates of this form of treatment. Nevertheless (except for some depressed patients) the majority of patients take part at some stage in reality orientation groups. The occupational therapist also plays an important part in the organization of games, musical events and other social activities which are designed to provide stimulation for patients as a part of their treatment.

Under the supervision of the occupational therapist the divisional therapist is particularly concerned with some of the social activities and also with a range of craft work. There is some division here between the sexes with female patients encouraged to knit, do needlework and make decorations while the male patients do elementary woodwork, sticking and glueing.

Within the hospital there is a widespread awareness of the importance of successful occupational therapy as part of an 'active therapeutic regime'. During one period in which no occupational therapist was in post the nursing staff themselves made considerable efforts to organize social and other diversional activities for patients although they complained repeatedly that they lacked the skill to do this.

Paramedical services

The day hospital is also serviced by a range of paramedical staff. These include a dietitian, physiotherapist, chiropodist, speech therapist and dentist.

The physiotherapist provides the equivalent of one 2.5-hour session per week for day-hospital patients. Day-hospital staff refer cases to the physiotherapist via the consultant psychiatrist. Of the cases in our six-month sample, only five are recorded as having received physiotherapy treatment. However, since each of the paramedical services keeps its own records about the patients which it treats and does not routinely put this information into the central medical files, this is almost certainly an underestimate. Nursing staff informed us that about 25% of patients are referred for physiotherapy.

The organization of chiropody services is a little different. The chiropodist is engaged for one 2.5-hour session each week organized as a half-hour per day for the day hospital. All patients are screened after admission and thereafter are seen at six-weekly intervals or more frequently if treatment is required. Again our estimate is that approximately 25% of patients get regular treatment additional to their six-weekly screening.

Likewise, the dietitian has one session per week for the day hospital. All patients are screened shortly after admission and a very high proportion of patients are assessed as having some dietary deficiency. Those needing treatment are referred to their GP via the medical officer. The day hospital does not systematically monitor treatment and operates primarily as a screening agent.

A speech therapy service is also available but patients are only seen following a specific request. Nursing staff explained that they themselves work with groups of dysphasic patients and that they use the speech therapist primarily as an adviser. In practice the service is a minor one within the day hospital.

Social work

We have already described the social worker's formal employment position. Essentially she undertakes three kinds of activities: first, assessment of patients' social background; second, coping with crises; and third, organizing the relatives' group. The social worker is rarely involved in 'therapy' or 'counselling' or any other form of direct treatment of patients. She does not, for example, undertake systematic group work with patients. Principally the social worker is concerned with relatives. Thus social work within the day hospital has the potential to influence the treatment of patients mainly by continual liaison between patients' relatives and the hospital. In practice, however, this does not occur as a routine matter. Rather, social work has adopted a reactive stance. (There is one significant exception: as we shall describe in Chapter 9 the social worker has played a major part in organizing the relatives' group.) At patient referral, a visit to the home to produce a social background report is made at the request of the consultant. Subsequent visits to relatives are usually at the request of either the psychiatrist or senior nursing staff when some problem connected with the patient's home arises. For example, on one occasion the social worker visited a patient at home at short notice when the patient was refusing to get on the bus. The nursing auxiliaries took the view that some discussion between the social worker and the relatives would be useful. Sometimes, too, the social worker calls on relatives if patients have not arrived in an attempt to find out why this has occurred. Although such activity may affect patients' attendance at the hospital, it does not usually take the form of direct contact between patients and social worker.

In short, although the social worker is held to provide an important service for this hospital, there are few areas in which social work service can be precisely identified as a contribution towards the 'active therapeutic regime' which is entailed in the treatment approach. There may be indirect benefits for the patients (and considerable benefits for medical staff) from social work activity in the day hospital but it is hard to relate it specifically to any improvement in their clinical condition.

Relatives attitudes towards the hospital services

We have now described the services through which attempts are made at the day hospital to cure patients. In presenting this description we have drawn upon our own observations, upon material we collected through the study of hospital records and upon accounts which staff themselves gave of the hospital services. Now we shall consider the attitudes of relatives towards services intended to treat and cure patients. These data provide another perspective on the clinical efficacy of the services.

Many relatives know very little about what actually happens to patients during the time that they spend in the day hospital and most relatives do not share the conception which staff have of a battery of assessment and therapeutic services focussing on patients' problems with a view to cure or significant improvement. For example:

> INTERVIEWER: 'Have you known enough of what actually happens at the day hospital, what he does and the kind of treatment he gets and things . . .?'
> MRS N: 'I really don't know what he gets – I know they try to get him to do things and I could hear from sister he's no very keen on complying with their ideas of trying to get him to do things but apart from that I really don't know what goes on.'

Some relatives can describe the range of services available but do so in rather general terms, probably from information routinely issued to patients at the time of admission. Even relatives who can list the services tend not to relate them to the treatment that their patient is receiving. There were even a few cases in which the relatives thought that the day hospital was making no treatment contribution additional to the prescriptions of the patient's GP.

> INTERVIEWER: 'What about the day hospital? Have you been able to find out what kind of treatment she's getting there or anything . . .?'
> MRS E: 'No, aw they're daein' is just gaein' her the tablets. They pills that she gets. That's a'. She's definitely worse the noo. She definitely is.'

(In many cases relatives were aware of the fact that they knew very little about the day hospital but they did not generally blame the institution for this. Most felt that the onus was on them to approach staff to find out about the patient, and the day hospital and its work. They saw the relatives' group as the forum for doing this and relatives who did not attend the group, for whatever reason, generally felt that the fault lay with them in not taking up the offer of consultation with staff.)

This lack of knowledge and the seeming lack of importance attached by relatives to the therapeutic services is rooted in their views about the reasons for the patient's admission to the day hospital in the first place and about the possibility of obtaining any cure. Relatives of patients suffering from dementia, in accord with their views about the condition generally, have little expectation of rehabilitation. (We discuss this point at much greater length in Chapter 9.) They tend to see the reasons for admission as relief for the family or as keeping the patient occupied. They place little emphasis upon the 'cure' of the patient. In the following example the relative was aware that such an opinion ran counter to that of the hospital staff but this did not change his view that the notion of a clinical cure was largely irrelevant to the patient's problems.

> INTERVIEWER: 'Do you think it is actually doing anything to help your mother?'
> MR K: 'No, well, doubtful, for I think she has gone beyond that stage. I mean I know the people out there probably don't but I feel myself that she has gone beyond the stage of rehabilitation or making her better than she is. I think she's beyond it. I saw too much deterioration in a short period to think that there's any way she'll ever be made any better than what she is. I very much doubt it. Being truthful.'

Not all relatives take exactly this view. Some are uncertain about prognosis and are concerned that there should be a possibility of improvement. Yet even they tend to be doubtful and are certainly not hopeful of a 'cure' as a result of day hospital intervention.

> INTERVIEWER: 'Did you think that the day hospital would actually be able to improve on her at all, on her condition?'
> MRS H: 'Its hard to say, because, if you've never had any dealin's wi' this kinna trouble before this kinna illness. I don't know whether there'd be room for improvement or no. I honestly don't know. I cannae see it. Maybe bodily wise, stronger, I cannae see how it could improve her mind, y'know. I really cannae see how it can improve, its mostly memory. I mean she cannae retain nothing. Its the memory. But I cannae see that they could help her memory. Other than they'd maybe make her dae things where I would say, "Och well, just leave it and I'll dae it for ye." – maybe that.'

It is not that relatives deny the benefits of treatment to patients but rather that they emphasize the importance of the day hospital as a source of company and activity. Some even rank this more highly than the medical benefits. As one relative said: '... but mainly I wasnae really concerned a great deal about the medical aspects of it, which was just to get her out and being active again.' In some cases relatives link lack of social activities with the cause of the patient's condition and therefore suggest that improvements, even if minor ones, might result if this deficiency is rectified. For others the provision of social activities is something simply to be valued in itself.

> INTERVIEWER: 'Did you think the day hospital might be able to do anything to make her any better?'
> MR H: 'No I didnae look at it on that line. Whit I looked at wis that she wis mixin' wi' people instead o' sittin' here a' week, she was getting' out twice a week to sit wi' these people, gettin' to know them and she was keepin' her mind interested – I widnae say active, but interested on people round about her, but – eh – making her better, no I don't think so. To me I'm under the impression that there's no – there'll never be any change, once agin I'll maybe be wrong, – eh – who am I to say I'm only the common layman and nobody – the doctors know better than me.'

Although the relatives of dementia patients (a majority of patients admitted to the day hospital) have little expectation of 'cure', some relatives of the minority of depressed patients have clearer hopes that the patient will improve as a result of attendance. But because of their higher expectations of patient improvement, these relatives also tend to have higher expectations of treatment and tend to be more critical of the service. As the relative of one depressed patient explained:

> INTERVIEWER: 'How do you see things going in the future?'
> MRS I: 'Well I would definitely hope they'd brighten. That's all I can say. But I'm wondering if she's needing some treatment that would be quicker.'
> INTERVIEWER: 'Do you not think that the hospital is offering much in the way of treatment?'
> MRS I: 'No, she's just getting exactly the same pills as she was getting sitting in that chair. She gets three Valium a day, you know that's what she gets on the Tuesday, she gets the same on the Wednesday. The only thing is she'll come home and say, "I knitted a coat hanger the day." And she could do that sitting in the chair if we were anxious but whether she would do it for us, I don't know.'

Although the hospital services do not generally operate as relatives would expect, that is not to say that they are ineffective. During interviews many relatives remarked that the patient had no regular contact with their own GP or that the GP's time or interest was limited. The day hospital may therefore compensate for the absence of the GP service in providing a general monitoring of the patient's condition by nursing staff, with medical back-up where necessary.

The form of treatment which relatives were most often able to point to was drug therapy. This was so particularly if drugs were taken in the form of injections administered at the day hospital. However, although relatives were more aware of this form of treatment than chiropody, occupational therapy or other forms of treatment, they again lacked any clear understanding of the nature and purposes of the medication. For example, several relatives said they knew that one commonly prescribed drug did not become very effective until after the third injection, but were confused about whether or not injections continued after the third dosage. They were also unsure about possible side effects.

This lack of knowledge of the details of medical treatment carried out at the day hospital (as of the services generally) was quite extensive. Relatives of one diabetic patient mentioned in interview that they did not know whether or not the day hospital conducted routine tests on the patient's sugar level. The relatives' group (as we shall see in Chapter 10) provided a setting in which some relatives could enquire about treatment. However, their enquiries underlined the way in which many were confused about the patient's medication even though relatives were themselves administering drugs to the patients.

So, to draw some conclusions on relatives' attitudes towards the hospital's services, our data indicate:

(1) widespread ignorance about the details of services;
(2) a rather critical approach on the part of some relatives; and
(3) a perspective on the possibility of patient improvement which is generally at variance with the idea of an active therapeutic regime.

We have said that these data do not in themselves indicate a lack of success as clinical cure. However, they do indicate a serious lack of involvement of relatives in any therapeutic programme which might be carried out in the home in conjunction with the day hospital. For example, we might expect that some of the techniques used in the day hospital could be successfully continued by relatives at home to reinforce any benefit experienced by the patient. Indeed some staff advocate such practice in general terms. Despite this, none of the relatives in our sample were involved in any such plans and very few even pointed to the day hospital as a source of advice on how best to handle the patient at home. As a final comment on the position of relatives, there is not any routine occasion on which relatives sit down with senior medical staff and take an overview of the patient's problems, treatment programme, prognosis and possible discharge.

Evidence on effectiveness

Let us recapitulate. The picture that is emerging of the day hospital's services is one in which patients are in receipt of a battery of separate therapies. Many of these are complements for inadequacies in services which they could be receiving elsewhere. Relatives are only marginally involved in the curative process. This is partly because there is divergence between relatives and hospital staff in the notions which they have of patients' problems and partly because of the way in which the hospital services are organized in a segmented way and without deliberate attention to the problems of integrating hospital and home support. In this section we shall ask if there is any further evidence, one way or the other, on the effectiveness of these services on the criterion of clinical cure. We shall look first at the hospital records and then at the Tuesday meetings.

Evidence in the records

In much of the literature on psychogeriatric care, as we discussed in Chapter 5, data on patient flow is in practice used to assess the effectiveness of a hospital's policies. Thus quite often discharges back to the community are treated as synonymous with clinical improvement. We have already argued that this is an unreliable equation. In examining our own six-month sample of cases, we have therefore taken a more detailed qualitative look at the case files of those patients discharged within our period of sample and follow-up. Of the total of forty-five admissions in this sample, nineteen cases manifestly deteriorated and were discharged either for long-term admission to a psychiatric hospital or to the care of some other institution as the result of either physical or mental deterioration, five cases were discharged either because the patient or the relatives refused to permit continued attendance, nine cases either died or became so seriously unfit as to be unable to attend the day hospital any further, five cases were still attending at the conclusion of our follow-up period, and on one case insufficient information exists to offer a classification. Of the remaining five cases one showed considerable reluctance to attend and was eventually discharged to the care of the community nurse, one was discharged to local authority day care after a period of assessment and one was 'discharged' onto a regime in which she attended the hospital every other month.

The two remaining cases are both described in the hospital records as discharged back to the community due to improved condition. One was a lady who had been admitted with the following comment from the psychiatrist:

> I suspected that Mrs H was a little forgetful but there was certainly no evidence of gross dementia. On the other hand she did seem a little depressed and there was a very strong paranoid flavour to her conversation. She might be someone we would help through the day hospital and arrangements have been made for her to have a trial period there attending on one day every week. I think we will take the opportunity of trying the effect of some sort of drug therapy and I hope it will be possible to bring about some improvement.

Her problem is diagnosed in the nursing report as paranoid psychosis, in the medical officer's report as 'chronic bronchitis, myocardiac insufficiency, obesity, degenerative arthritis of the spine, and depression', and in the nursing care plan as 'delusional, paranoid, manipulative and having a mobility problem'. She was a patient of the hospital for some 2.5 months and was discharged after the following comments in the nursing report.

> 22.7 Social work assistant asked to visit to assess home condition with a view to discharge.
> 24.7 Visited by social work assistant. Patient would appear to be coping very well at home but is developing a reliance on [the day hospital].
> 6.8 Patient now reached obtainable level of independence. Progress good. Discharged into the community.

The medical officer commented: 'Discharged from day hospital. But unlikely to improve further.' Although in this case hospital staff took the view that the patient had improved significantly during her stay at the hospital, there is no quantified material in the hospital records which permits independent verification of that judgement.

The second case 'discharged to the community' was admitted after a psychiatric report stating that 'the clinical symptom and symptomatology is in keeping with a bereavement reaction. I am making arrangements with the community psychiatric staff to visit her and arrange a place in the day hospital.' The social background report reads:

> Condition at present according to the son is improving. He still feels that a period of day care would help to reintroduce his mother into society again (after the bereavement). Therefore I would recommend a period of one month's assessment to be offered at this time to Mrs K.

The nursing report records the immediate problem as 'recently bereaved'. The patient was admitted to the hospital for two periods, one lasting almost three months and the second, some three months later, lasting almost six months. In the middle of the second period a monthly discharge regime was started and eventually she was discharged with the following nursing report:

> Reattended today after a month's discharge. Offers no complaints. Discussed at Conference. Discharged to community due to improved mental and physical state. Attends social clubs in community.

Crichton scaling was completed over both periods, on the first occasion moving from a score of sixteen to fourteen to sixteen over three weeks and on the second occasion moving from a score of 18.5 to eighteen over four weeks. The final Crichton assessment was made some two months before the date of final discharge. Again, although this patient is assessed as having improved, there is apparently little quantified data upon which this judgement was based.

It is this kind of detailed inspection of clinical files which indicates why caution is so necessary in equating discharge with clinical improvement. Our most optimistic conclusion must be that, of the forty-five admissions in our sample, two have significantly improved and this clinical improvement may be due to attendance at the day hospital. A more pessimistic conclusion would be that hard evidence on clinical improvement is not available for any of the forty-five cases. At best the active therapeutic regime of the hospital is having a significant effect on 5% of the cases admitted.

There is a major qualification that we should enter to this argument. It might be suggested that although the day hospital does not, apparently, effect a significant 'cure' it does slow down the rate at which patients deteriorate (especially those eventually admitted to permanent care). This is an important argument which is closely related to our discussion of patient flow. But although this is a very plausible suggestion for the small number of patients who stay for a lengthy period, it cannot be claimed as a significant consequence for the much higher proportion of patients who remain in the hospital for only a brief period. Ironically, the very success of the day hospital in maintaining a throughput of patients and avoiding 'silt up' is evidence of the fact that it does not act as a long-term stabilizing influence upon patients who would otherwise deteriorate. Generally, institutions of this kind which 'silt up,' as we discussed in Chapter 5, are regarded as failures since their inability to discharge patients is taken as evidence of their inability to effect a cure. That argument can be turned on its head. Broadly speaking (and to judge from the records), this day hospital is achieving a rapid throughput of patients, with little evidence of their having improved, and with a high proportion of them passing quickly to long-term care.

Evidence in the meetings

So far in this section we have placed considerable emphasis on the availability of quantified and recorded material as the basis for assessing patients. (This reflects the emphasis of the 'treatment model'.) However, such an approach should not be allowed to obscure the potential validity of assessment made without recorded quantifiable data by professional staff in close and regular contact with the patients. Therefore, in order to see whether or not such assessment of clinical improvement is used as a basis for discharging patients, we inspected our transcripts of Tuesday meetings and our field notes on these occasions to see if there was sound evidence on the criterion of clinical cure available from these discussions which was not apparent within the patients' files and records.

We have already presented some lengthy extracts from our transcripts of Tuesday meetings and have described the way in which admission decisions are made. The discussions surrounding discharge decisions are typically much briefer and contain significantly less information about patients. The following is a conversation which preceded the possible discharge of Mrs K, one of the two 'success' stories that we described above:

> SISTER: 'Mrs K came in – can we try her on the monthly discharge regime [name of consultant]? I think she is latching on to the department.'
> CONSULTANT: 'Did we do this before with her?'
> SISTER: 'No, we discharged her before and then got her rereferred but I thought . . .'
> CONSULTANT: 'Was she from a nursing home in A?'
> SISTER: 'No.'
> COMMUNITY NURSE: 'One of Dr T's patients. We had her in a short time and discharged her and had to take her back in and then she was discharged again and they wanted her to attend . . .'
> CONSULTANT: 'O.K.? Will somebody keep an eye on her . . .?'
> COMMUNITY NURSE: 'Uhu.'
> SISTER: 'Uhu. Uhu. I'll pass her on to the community . . .'
> CONSULTANT: 'Because these are the ones that sometimes . . .'
> COMMUNITY NURSE: 'She's not on the [trade name of drug].'
> SISTER: 'No.'
> COMUNITY NURSE: 'I visited her before you know.'
> CONSULTANT: 'We sometimes had problems with this . . .' [The discussion moves to the next case.]

Of course it is not only at the point of discharge that the clinical progress of a case is discussed. As we have described, sister introduces discussion on a number of cases on the basis of the nursing notes at Tuesday meetings when time allows. It is possible that these discussions form the basis of a discharge decision and a clinical picture of the case may build up from week to week through these discussions. The following is an illustration of one such discussion at a Tuesday meeting:

SISTER: 'Mrs G. That was the wee lady last week. You got the letter about her as well, about attacking the home help. Dr P contacted you.'
CONSULTANT: 'Oh! yes. With the poker, yes.'
SISTER: 'We brought her in five days a week. She's no problem and we've got the poker. What do you want me to do with the poker?' [Laughter]
COMMUNITY NURSE: 'Tie it in a knot and give it her back!'
SISTER: 'Use it on the . . .'
CONSULTANT: 'Hm . . .'
SISTER: 'She's no trouble in here [name of consultant]. I think maybe its flared up between the home help and herself. I don't think she's ever been any trouble. She gets agitated but she wants to go home. She doesn't even do that now she's quite settled.'
NURSE: 'Her house she keeps it quite well. And she does washing. She saw the previous home help as interfering, going through her drawers and cupboards and what not, as a criticism of herself, y'know, and probably resents the fact that this woman is coming in and . . .'
SISTER: 'She still has a coal fire and I'm wondering what she's using to poke the fire with, y'know ... if she starts using a piece of wood or something like that you've got a danger set up.'
CONSULTANT: 'Yes. Dr N phoned me. I think he had the home help supervisor in the room with him . . .'
SISTER: 'That's Mrs K. She was terrible when she phoned here.'
CONSULTANT: '... Twisting his arm. Hm – so I don't really know what his own views are.'
SISTER: 'Well she said that Dr H had said to take the home help home and charge Mrs G. Now we work with Dr H in the hospital and he's in our own practice and I can't imagine him saying THAT. I mean, Mrs K said that Dr H advised that she went to the police and charged Mrs G. I mean she's 83 years old goodness sake, and she's a wee frail thing, its not as if she's a big terrible hulk or anything.'
CONSULTANT: 'Hmm . . . I couldn't imagine Dr H saying that . . .'
SISTER: 'We said that ... that it was an emergency, that's why she was up to five days, but the feeling is Mrs K won't let us reduce her [days of attendance], she'll put up an awful fight if she's going to reduce at all.'
CONSULTANT: 'Its incredible though what people say that their doctors have said to them. Most of the time when you advise people they take it or leave it as they wish but sometimes it suits them to not only take it but to embroider it a bit.'
SISTER: 'I think its been used because she's demanding a bed and she wanted yourself to put it in writing that Mrs G, y'know, was a danger in the community and I said to her, "Oh! well, its not [the consultant's] policy to put it in writing, anything in writing" to home helps or anybody.'
CONSULTANT: [Laughing].
SISTER: 'I didn't say that! I mean she wanted this in black and white that this woman was an emergency case and that she was attacking . . .'
COMMUNITY NURSE: 'Who is this K?'
SISTER: [Gives christien name] 'K. Home-help organizer in [nearby town].'
CONSULTANT: 'Hm?'

SISTER: 'She was demanding a bed . . .'
NURSE: 'She goes shopping . . . I mean she came to us twice a week and those three days she went out and did shopping and did her washing and the house is clean; she builds a fire. And y'know it would be a shame to put that woman in a bed even supposing there were . . .'
SISTER: 'I said to her that she's not one of our emergencies but "She is an emergency!" but I said, "She's not one of our emergencies – all the emergencies are on the waiting list." No way. And she came out with Dr H said this woman was to be charged by the police and I thought, "Oh well, you're just obviously threatening." I couldn't imagine Dr H saying it because he would have to contact here first or yourself first because he is in our practice.'
NURSE: 'Plus it's [the medical officer] and I mean he's in the same practice and he came in and he said, "Oh! no." Dr H wouldn't have said that.'
OCCUPATIONAL THERAPIST: 'I haven't been able to assess her as far as kitchen work is concerned because when I broached the subject with her she got – hm – quite adamant that she coped very well and there was no need to do anything like that with me here.'
SISTER: 'She does. I mean she helped her with the dishes, etc., y'know.'
OTHERS: 'Yes that's right.' [Confirmation from all sides.]
CONSULTANT: 'Well what she doesn't [inaudible] with the poker!' [General laughter]
OCCUPATIONAL THERAPIST: 'I mean she just walked away from me. That was quite a . . . that was the situation when she could have stood . . . been nasty . . . she just walked away.'
SISTER: 'She's never been aggressive in here at all.'
NURSE: 'She's never . . . the personality of the home help.'
SISTER: 'There may have been a clash. She's gone in and there's been a clash.'
CONSULTANT: 'Well – hm – again I think when [the social worker] returns this is one we'll have to ask her to work on, not specifically Mrs G . . .'
SISTER: 'Mrs K.' [Laughter]
CONSULTANT: 'So . . . but . . . can you continue her five days?'
SISTER: 'Oh! yes. Uhu.'
CONSULTANT: 'O.K.'

The importance of this extract for our present concern is that, although there is some debate about the patient's condition, a substantial proportion of the discussion is about the attitudes of another agency (in this case the home-help service) towards the patient and the hospital. There is apparently little attempt to systematically measure the patient's clinical performance. A further extract illustrates discussion at the Tuesday meeting surrounding a larger number of cases, some of which were being considered for discharge:

CONSULTANT: 'Miss D. Eh? Anything to say about her?'
SISTER: 'No, she's in the department. She's actually coming back to the department now. Its just this holiday admission that they're requesting in.'
CONSULTANT: 'Mr E not coming?'
SISTER: 'He's still not coming. He said last week he wouldn't . . . [The social worker] went out as well, but she couldn't get in the house either.'
SOCIAL WORKER: 'Well I think that was . . . it was a bit early of course and they may have been in their bed. But they're not letting anybody in.'
SISTER: 'The daughter phoned up and said that he had put on half a stone in

weight and doesn't need to go back to this department. But – eh – really she was saying no as well as he's saying no.'

CONSULTANT: 'Well we won't waste any more time on Mr E. If he changes his mind later.'

SOCIAL WORKER: '. . . his wife doing this daft . . .'

CONSULTANT: 'Well you can drop them a note. Mrs F.'

SISTER: 'Mrs F has been admitted to the [local authority home] for two weeks holiday admission . . .'

CONSULTANT: 'Oh!'

SISTER: '. . . the day after you were there you said he phoned up and said she was coming back and then the husband phoned up in the morning to say that she would be admitted to the [home] on the 15th and she'd phone when she came back out . . . the 15th, last week.'

CONSULTANT: 'Mrs N?'

COMMUNITY NURSE: 'She's back, yes.'

CONSULTANT: 'Oh! the one with the . . .'

SISTER: 'Not dying at all. Full of beans.'

COMMUNITY NURSE: 'She was O.K. when I saw her last week.'

SISTER: 'I think the daughter is most peculiar y'know, she really is, I mean she was in yesterday and she seen chiropody and now the daughter says there's no change in her feet and has she seen the chiropodist. I don't know what changes she's expecting though but . . .'

COMMUNITY NURSE: 'The daughter went upstairs when I went in . . .'

SISTER: '. . . she's full of beans and [the medical officer] examined her for the fall.'

COMMUNITY NURSE: 'The old lady says – eh [whispers] "They've got me well insured, they jist want rid o' me. They jist want rid o' me that's all." It's rather a queer household that.'

CONSULTANT: 'K.T. She – eh – I think I saw her sitting there this morning.'

SOCIAL WORKER: 'She's really . . . a worry.'

OCCUPATIONAL THERAPIST: 'I haven't seen her this week. The kitchen practice. I'll try and see her next week.'

CONSULTANT: 'O.K. Mrs K.'

SISTER: 'Mrs K, we got a phone call last week from the police asking if we had Mrs K in here on Tuesday morning; she had absconded from the home at half-past seven and was not found till half-past eleven and the husband is as confused as she is – I think because he didn't know where she was when he had last seen her or anything and the son telephoned as well, but the police phoned back to let us know she was found at half-past eleven so we . . . she's settled in well in the department and she's lucid on the surface – but again underneath –'

OCCUPATIONAL THERAPIST: 'I had a long chat with her and she said this about her mother coming.'

CONSULTANT: 'Yes – hm – that's right.'

SISTER: 'But – eh – I'm worried about the husband . . . well because we can't really get much from him because he's very confused as well.

CONSULTANT: 'Yes I think I knew that the husband was in question though not as bad as his wife.'

SOCIAL WORKER: 'I think that – hm – he's functional in that he can go out and buy things and appear to be O.K. but I think he's not very *reliable* – eh – in helping with her y'know, I don't think he would be any help at all, it's really the son that'll keep things, and the home help and district nurse they all kind of go in.'

CONSULTANT: 'Mrs Q – we've spoken about Ann D.'

SISTER: 'Ann D is now in [a general hospital].'

CONSULTANT: 'Is she?'
SISTER: 'She was transferred there. The Infirmary telephoned us.'
CONSULTANT: 'I wondered why I haven't heard any more from the Infirmary.'
SISTER: 'Plus she developed a chest infection and she's been taken out to Dr K's Unit. I don't know, we might get pressure from them.'
SOCIAL WORKER: 'Very very confused apparently.'
SISTER: 'He's a bit better I think ...'

In this extract both the brevity of discussion on each case and the absence of supportive evidence are very striking.

Maintaining the reality of 'an active therapeutic regime'

In this chapter we have been examining the extent to which the range of day hospital services which we have described operate in a way which is consistent with a 'treatment model'. We have concluded that much of what takes place in connection with the clinical treatment of patients cannot be explained as consistent with this approach and that there is little evidence to suggest that the day hospital is successful in treating its patients in these terms. Other variables and social processes are operative.

Nevertheless, as we have demonstrated both in this chapter and in greater detail in Chapter 4, a sense of achieving an effective therapeutic regime is central to the culture of the day hospital. In this final section, therefore, we shall suggest how it is that this 'culture of cure' is actively maintained. For this institution is geared to preserving an image and reputation of 'success', sometimes at least in the face of evidence to the contrary.

Our comments below are divided into two sections. The first deals with the way in which the institution as a whole is regarded as successful on the criterion of clinical cure. The second outlines the way in which a definition of successful treatment is assigned to particular individual patients in discussions between staff, and in discussions between staff and relatives.

A successful institution

First, then, we deal with the way in which an image of success is sustained for the institution as a whole.

(1) SELECTIVE QUOTATION There is the use of selective quotation. Although for the majority of patients, as we have discussed, 'cure' is improbable if not impossible, staff can point selectively to the fact that for *some* patients there is *some* improvement on at least *some* count. As a psychiatrist explained:

INTERVIEWER: 'You have said that it's [senile dementia] an irreversible process. I wonder what implications that has for the day hospital in terms of the treatment that can be offered to these patients?'
CONSULTANT: '... but of course not all our patients coming to the day hospital are dementias, mind you. Some of them are confusional states which are potentially reversible and some of them are depressions and paranoid states and so on which can be improved.'

And there are always some instances of improvement which staff can refer to in support of the general view that patients do improve. As one nurse explained:

> We have had two patients in that have been termed psychogeriatric and we've said, 'Well, they really need a bed', but you know there isn't a bed, so we take them in. They have the medication stopped. These patients are back out now in the community and you ought to see them going shopping etc. Now that's really great, you know they are like that. If there had been a bed and this place hadn't been here, the future for them would have been that they would have been psychogeriatric . . .

This potential for selective quotation is generally facilitated by the way in which, as we have shown, there is no unambiguous statement of 'the problem' to start with.

The potential for selective quotation is also facilitated by the way in which the day hospital is segmented into a series of separate services. Sometimes it is difficult to make detailed links between services. For example, we have described the way in which the separate professions tend to keep their own records on specific treatments in relation to the specific problems with which they are particularly concerned. On occasions this means that nursing, social work, or other staff may quite accurately see an improvement in the condition of the patients with respect to some particular facet of the problem and may conclude from this that an assessment of improvement overall is justified. Yet from a more detached perspective any such judgement would have to be qualified substantially. We have also explained that very different pictures of the patient are inclined to emerge from their home and from the hospital. Relatives point out that the assessment which nursing staff make of the patient on the basis of their behaviour within the hospital is only a partial perspective on the patient's overall condition.

(2) RITUALS The culture of cure is reinforced by ritualistic adherence to some of the day hospital systems. We have discussed the use of the Crichton scaling rates and have shown how the practical use of this system of assessment differs from the planned ideal. The operational policies of the day hospital contain a number of such systems. For example there are arrangements for nurses to meet in teams and discuss the nursing care plans of particular patients. Again, we have found considerable difficulty in relating the detailed strategies outlined in these plans to the practical decisions about discharge and variations in treatment. In the absence of firm evidence of clinical improvement for the vast majority of patients, adherence to the rituals of formal arrangements becomes a substitute for clinical effectiveness.

(3) ASSESSMENT The way in which the notion of assessment is used fosters the culture of cure. Patients are very often admitted to the day hospital for a 'period of assessment'. So far as the practical treatment of the patients is concerned, there is little difference between those attending the hospital for assessment and those who have been admitted as cases for treatment. Nevertheless the notion of a patient being assessed allows staff to avoid confronting the fact that

the treatment is having little effect. May and Smith (1980) have described the way in which assessment is used in the field of juvenile justice to evade the known fact that many delinquency programmes produce no measurable improvement in the behaviour of delinquents. A similar process seems to be at work in this institution. Through the notion of assessment professionals delay, sometimes indefinitely, the specific point in the career of the patient at which a decision on the efficacy of treatment must be made.

(4) PATIENT FLOW A culture of cure is fostered by confusing curative practices and the flow of patients through the day hospital. We have discussed this point at some length already in this chapter and pointed out that the two should not be equated. But a notion of failure is not readily available within a medical institution and the fact that staff generally deny the possibility of discharging cases that have deteriorated explains the tendency to equate discharges with cases of clinical improvement. The following extract from one of our interviews illustrates the point. A senior nurse is speaking:

> ... if in the course of time you are able to discharge them, it is obvious that they have improved enough to be discharged. I don't, as I recollect, think that we have ever discharged anyone that we haven't been able to help back to their own home on their own, y'know, or if they have regretted it in any way I can't recollect a specific case where we have done that, because I think this, this would be an unacceptable practice ...

The practice of intermittent readmission can also be used to sustain an image of success where permanent discharge is not achieved. At each discharge a sense of optimism prevails and, so far as the general perspective on the day hospital is concerned, overshadows the readmissions which intervene.

(5) A SPECIALITY Finally it is always possible for staff to explain away apparent clinical failures by pointing to the fact that they can cope only with psychiatric problems and a patient may well deteriorate either because of complications in their social background or because of physical deterioration. While in some contexts it is claimed to be an important feature of the day hospital that it provides a social-work and a general medical service as well as a psychiatric service, on other occasions staff revert to a more narrow definition of the day hospital's major functions and describe it primarily as a psychogeriatric hospital.

Successful cases

In describing success in clinical practice, staff are inclined to refer to the workings of the day hospital as a whole. In this way specific cases of deterioration are obscured. There are occasions, however, when staff must confront the fact that some individual patients have not improved. Sometimes this confrontation occurs in interaction between staff and sometimes in interaction between staff and relatives. In both settings the significance of little or no improvement is minimized.

Between staff we might expect some consideration of failure to occur at discharge when the patient is not returning home (the vast majority of cases) and, particularly, when the patient is being admitted to long-term care. As we have seen, the incentive to discharge is strong and the material that we have already presented in this chapter shows how brief, for the most part, is the detailed consideration of the case at the point of discharge. The brevity of this discussion simply means that the deteriorating aspects of the case are just not discussed.

Similarly, the decision to admit a patient to long-term care is not considered in a way which implies failure. The fact that the patient has probably deteriorated significantly is outweighed by other considerations which give rise to a sense of satisfaction. First, long-term beds and places in long-term residential care are extremely difficult to obtain. There is some sense of achievement that a place has become available and that the consultant has been successful in obtaining it for a day hospital patient. Generally staff are also pleased that they have been able to delay, as they see it, admission to a long-term bed for as long as they have. Failing all else, staff can return to the notion that senile dementia is essentially an irreversible process and that the day hospital has been as successful as possible. It could not have been expected to have achieved any more. The culture of therapy in this field is ambiguous. It moves between a view of the merits of actively pursuing a therapeutic regime while nevertheless adhering on occasions to the view that the condition is irreversible.

Some features of the process of maintaining a culture of success with respect to individual patients are also apparent in interaction between staff and relatives. It has been evident in our discussions of relatives' views of the 'problem', of the services of the day hospital, and of the effectiveness of treatment, that for the majority of relatives clinical cure is not a reality. However, since most relatives have very little contact with staff their different perspectives on 'curing' the patient give rise to little conflict.

The exception to this observation is the relatives' group, which is attended by a minority of patients' relatives and which does provide a forum where negotiation between the two perspectives takes place. There are several ways in which staff sustain the notion of patient improvement here. They can always quote minor non-specific improvements such as 'he's settling' or 'she's brighter today'. Staff may quote improvements occurring at the day hospital where relatives experience no similar improvement in the home. Staff may also quote specific facets of patient behaviour which have been assessed at the day hospital and which have shown improvements even though these are not the behaviours with which the relatives are experiencing greatest difficulty. A further tactic is to compare patients, one with another, pointing to the fact that although a particular problem may not have been overcome in one case it has been in a comparable case. In cases where staff have difficulty in producing examples of improvement and where relatives are persistent in pointing to deterioration, the staff may use a 'period of assessment' which the patient is undergoing as the reason for lack of effective action in the meantime. Staff may also resort to technical explanations of why something is happening or point out that 'it is to be expected' in a way that effectively terminates the interchange.

Although we deal with interaction between staff and relatives in greater detail in Chapters 9 and 10, the following extract from the transcript of a relatives' group illustrates some of the points that we have just made:

> MRS M: '... Eh, as I say, just about these hallucinations, this is the worrying bit, he can manage fine other than that, he manages fairly well.'
> SISTER: 'Yes the OT had him in the kitchen and that, she's trying to get him away from the frying pan and get him on to more convenience foods like mashed [potato powder], cans, things that he can open that he doesn't have to put in the frying pan, and maybe get burnt in the kitchen. And he made a cheese and potato pie and sat down and ate it. It was lovely too.'
> MRS M: 'He's great ...'
> NURSE: 'His medication's changed anyway ...'
> MRS M: 'I phoned, when I couldn't manage the last time, about that to see if you could do something.'
> SISTER: 'It might be tomorrow though, because he was on it for a week and it was a week's reviews, so [the consultant] will review it tomorrow and see ... but certainly the hallucinations haven't altered.'
> MRS M: 'They haven't altered. And still seem to be having trouble during the night, again I live in [a nearby town] but, eh, the immediate neighbours on one side and the back of him have been saying that he's going out and about at night till the early hours of the morning. Again they're hearing a lot of noises but I'm quite sure this is what it is, because you know ... these people and a lot of swearing, a thing you never heard him do before is swear, he never ever swore. But he eats well, he eats more than my husband can eat and when he's at home he's got a tremendous appetite and he copes very well with his cooking. You've a bother to get him to change his clothes, eh, that's a problem but as far as washing or shaving goes, no problem there.'

Conclusion

A general theme running through this chapter refers to what we might call the dangers of the diversionary ideal. We began by describing some of the difficulties of a strictly clinical model in day care for the elderly mentally infirm. In particular there is no unambiguous definition of the 'problem'. We have described the services which the day hospital offers to its patients and we have attempted an evaluation of the success of these services on the criterion of clinical cure – in part by drawing upon relatives' interpretations but (perhaps more importantly) by drawing also upon the evidence which the day hospital itself marshals in relation to its own practices. Our conclusion has been that the clinical model leaves much to be explained in the organization of day hospital services. In a final section we described how staff maintain an ideology of successful clinical practice in spite of a good deal of evidence suggesting that the success of the day hospital on this count is rather limited. Our comment on the practical implications of this process is that the day hospital may be failing to do some things which it could do rather well because it continues to pursue an ideal which it is not likely to achieve. That is what we mean by the danger of the diversionary ideal. An analysis of what the day hospital may realistically achieve must be the subject of other chapters in which we approach its services from the standpoint of alternative criteria of success.

CHAPTER SEVEN

Success as Integrated Service

Introduction

Most day hospitals for the elderly mentally infirm offer a variety of medical, psychiatric and social services to patients, and staff consider this variety to be an important aspect of the hospital's success.

Goldstein et al. (1968), for example, describe one psychogeriatric day hospital (see also Goldstein et al. 1975 and Goldstein and Carlson 1976). They pay particular attention to the way in which it is staffed by psychiatrists, part-time medical and psychiatric residents, registered nurses, a social worker, and a group worker. An occupational therapist assesses functional capabilities, a psychologist undertakes testing and group therapy and a part-time general practitioner deals with physical illness. All these staff generally attend a weekly ward meeting. The psychiatrist is head of the team but a 'team leader' (nurse) is responsible for the day-to-day functioning of the hospital, and team members (with the exception of the psychiatrist) actually carry out most of the direct work with patients. Although there is some discrepancy in views between the psychiatrist and team members, and although there is some ambiguity in the roles of some staff, a sense of successful operation is maintained because of a prime loyalty of all staff to the team. Indeed, so clear is this perception on the part of staff that even though 'after one year of operation we have not had a single discharge as a result of patient improvement', 'the need for the type of service we provide seems obvious to us' (1968, p. 958). Goldstein et al. (1968, p. 958) conclude this account with the following comment:

> Having so many diagnostic and treatment resources centralized is not only convenient for the patients, but also makes hospital facilities available to a large number of patients. We believe that we are able to support people in the community who might otherwise be in psychiatric wards or in nursing homes.

Goldstein's account is quite typical (cf. Berger and Berger 1971). Wadsworth et al. (1972) describe a geriatric day hospital which entails the services of occupational therapy, physiotherapy, medical, social-work and chiropody, as well as medical and dental staff. A nursing sister fills a key role in the organization of day-to-day events. Although there is a problem of the consultant overriding GPs and the social worker, and resisting the team approach, this is explained as a function of insecurity. McDonald et al. (1971) describe a team in which 'all staff members except the psychiatrist, physician and secretary, work as individual therapists and have primary responsibility for the geriatric patients assigned to them' (p. 323). The account by Greiff and McDonald (1973) of the roles of staff in a psychogeriatric day centre is largely consistent with that of Goldstein, noting, in particular, the team approach as a major factor in the success of the unit. The value attached to the team approach mirrors the value which is placed on team work in related services also – for example, in the care of the terminally ill (see: Working Group on Terminal Care 1980; Bates et al. 1981; Thomas 1982).

The picture that emerges, then, is this. Day hospitals for the elderly mentally infirm typically entail the provision of a range of psychiatric, medical, social work and associated services. The precise list varies between hospitals but it is unusual not to contain psychiatric consultancy, medical services (often of a part-time GP), nursing, occupational therapy, physiotherapy, and social work. The services of a specialized group worker, dietitian or psychologist and the availability of in-patient beds are more variable features (cf. Peace 1980).

The staff involved in the provision of these services work as a team. This feature of the work of the day hospital is widely held to improve the quality of services and is therefore advanced as a most important measure of the success of the institution. Usually all senior staff attend a weekly case conference/staff meeting and participate fully in major decisions about admissions, discharges and operational policies. This meeting, amongst other activities, generates an *esprit de corps* amongst staff which in turn generates a perception of successful functioning. Although this form of organization may involve a broadening of the role of some practitioners and some role ambiguity and uncertainty, such confusion is regarded as minor and soluble through clarification. The working of the team entails a notion of the equal part that all members play within the day hospital (although, in practice, traditional medical hierarchies of authority and control are seldom far away – in particular, the consultant psychiatrist remains, in law and practice, in charge). The consultant typically relies heavily upon a senior nurse who effectively works as the day-to-day team leader and is a kind of 'first lieutenant' to the consultant. The consultant relies upon the nurse for information and the nurse upon the consultant for authority to guide the team. As well as co-ordinating separate facets of the day hospital services, such arrangements are deemed to improve communication both between staff members and with relatives and patients.

Thus, overall, the organization, co-ordination and provision of a range of professional services through team work is itself regarded as a mark of a successful service. It is one of the central distinguishing features of a 'day hospital', as opposed to out-patient clinic, day-care centre or social club.

The day hospital in our study is quite typical in these respects. Throughout the early phase of planning and establishing the hospital, the organization and provision of a range of services through a team of professionals was regarded as a most significant feature of the institution. There was much concern that it should not be merely a 'glorified luncheon club'. This meant that patients should spend a significant amount of time in attendance each day and that the hospital should provide a comprehensive medical and social service to meet a wide range of patients' needs. During the course of making staff appointments, drawing up operational policies, and overseeing the initial phase of the development, the establishment of social work and paramedical services were a focus of particular attention.

It is true that there was some confusion about the roles that some members of staff should occupy. For example, an occupational therapist arrived, suggesting that she should carry out home visits on a routine basis. She was met with the objection that this practice would encroach upon community services and that it would take her away from the hospital. Although the social worker was intended to be a member of the team, no accommodation was provided for her in the day hospital. (After much negotiation she was provided with an office in the Park Hospital buildings.) Senior nursing staff also objected on occasions to their lack of control over the social worker since she was employed by the local authority social work department. There were also difficulties in staff recruitment aggravated by the fact that a number of auxiliary services – not only social work – were not under direct working-party control. Speech therapy, dietetics, occupational therapy and dentistry were all on occasions difficult to sustain.

Nevertheless, the organization and provision of a range of integrated services through the work of a team of professionals is widely advanced by staff and administrators as one of the major criteria of success by which the work of the day hospital should be evaluated. Moreover, there is a general sense within the day hospital that its services rank highly on this count. The provision of a range of services by a team of professionals is valued in itself and a strong commitment to the team ideal, good interprofessional communication, and the opportunity for participation and shared decision-making – all resulting in improved service provision – are advanced as the main aspects of this ideal.

We can quote from our interviews to illustrate these points. The consultant that we quoted in Chapter 6 (p. 83) explained that the day hospital delivers a wide range of services and that this is what distinguishes it from a 'day' or 'social centre':

> Well – hm – treatment that wouldn't be offered in a social centre? Yes – hm – we can certainly in the day hospital look at the question of drugs, can't we? ... Of course they can't that in a social centre. We can offer occupational therapy in the sense of assessment and training as opposed to diversional. Then physiotherapy ... it's often more convenient to do so and, as you know, the physiotherapist attends the weekly meeting and incidentally provides some kind of link with physiotherapy services outside. Diet, – there's a number of our patients who I think have

developed confusional states or at least where confusion has added to the dementia if you like, through inadequate diet and we can, when we have a dietitian make some kind of assessment of what the patient's diet really is and then try to correct any deficiences one way or another. Chiropodist – of course we've got – and there again we have quite a few problems with feet. Again these can be dealt with outside the day hospital but sometimes it's more convenient to do so in this setting ... so we've got a medical aspect to it. Physiotherapy, occupational therapy, chiropody, diet, nursing care of course in a general sort of way, that can help too. So these are all things we can offer which a day centre can't.

However, it is not merely the availability of a range of services which is important but also the integration of the various professions in a team approach to patients' problems. Staff place great stress on the value of good teamwork as several respondents explained – for example, a community nurse:

Well, as I say, I think the very important thing is that the team aspect of the whole approach ... we felt that this was y'know, the only way to get ... you must have *harmony* because you're working with a team and you don't want one member pulling at another, I think we were mature enough to know that and realize that from the outset that it's O.K. if we work as a team we'll get something done.

Central to the development of good teamwork is the need for staff to meet together and discuss patients. The weekly Tuesday meeting provides the main arena for this and staff are strongly committed to this meeting both as an essential feature of the operation of the day hospital and as a means of promoting good interdisciplinary communication:

INTERVIEWER: 'A specific area that it might be quite interesting to talk about is the Tuesday meeting and how you see that in the operation of the day hospital.' NURSE: 'I think it's very useful, I think it would be tragic if we didn't have it. The place wouldn't function as it does if we didn't have the regular Tuesday meeting. I'm very glad that [the consultant] puts his emphasis on that, he doesn't like anyone not to be at that meeting at all. Come hell, rain or whatever you must be at that meeting on a Tuesday apart from when you are on holiday or if you are off sick. I think it is *very* important, I think it's the only time that the whole team can get together as one unit and discuss the patient.'

A social worker also explained;

... the most important thing is that we actually have a team meeting weekly and that is never allowed to go – hm – I think that's the one thing that builds [good communication] up – hm – I think the major people, the main people, like sister and myself – eh – [the psychiatrist, community nurse and senior enrolled nurse] y'know are always at these meetings – hm – therefore that ... that's the nub, that's the thing that keeps it going, that's where the whole communication comes from, all the other things are important but they're not the thing that keeps it going.

However, as a nurse explained, Tuesday meetings do not necessarily allow everyone to express a view in decision-making:

... I think this is one of our strong points, that a patient or somebody can be discussed openly and you can say how you feel, there's nothing held against you, you can say how you feel, but as I say it doesn't come to a vote on it, really ... I mean you express an opinion ... but that gentleman [i.e. the consultant] is the man who makes ... I mean if we say we don't think he's suitable and HE says he is suitable, well – he'll come in, you know. But this is how I feel about the Tuesday meeting, everyone can ... you've got the opportunity to put your piece in, how you feel about a situation, how you think it should be handled, whether right or wrong, I mean, as I say, nobody'll sort of pillory you first for it, and to me it is one of the great strengths of the hospital and the Tuesday meeting is very, very important.

Although staff value teamwork in its own right, they also claim that it improves services by increasing co-ordination within the Health Service and between health and social-work services. As we have noted (p. 47), a community nurse explained:

We're getting a greater liaison going with all the services, that it's not nearly as hard now when you phone up for a GP, or a home help or a clinic or a health visitor, they know through the centre, through the day hospital, what we're after and how much we can help and how much they can help us. I think ... its a focal point to bring all the services together ...

And a psychiatrist stressed the benefits of the team making social-work referals:

... outwith [the day hospital] you can still – eh – refer this to the social services but believe me there's a world of difference between speaking to [the social worker] with whom you've worked for quite a long time and speaking on the telephone to somebody you've never seen, in fact, well, I'll leave it at that! [Laughing].

The patient, it is claimed, also benefits:

INTERVIEWER: 'Is there some particular advantage for the patient in getting these services within a day hospital setting rather than, for example, as out-patients?' MEDICAL OFFICER: 'Yes, well all services can be co-ordinated, for example if I try to arrange chiropody as a GP I may have to wait three months, for other services it may be six months.'

So, from the start of this day hospital, although there were difficulties in sustaining some resources, although there was some ambiguity about the roles of some staff, and although some authority relations within the team remained ambiguous, the provision of a co-ordinated range of services was regarded as significant and staff were buoyed up in their enthusiasm for the hospital by a sense of being and working in a 'team' and providing a 'whole' service to patients and relatives. Moreover there was the strong sense that on this criterion of evaluation the day hospital is a success.

In the rest of this chapter we shall set this ideal against some further data on the day-to-day operation and functions of the day hospital. The problem with the picture of the day hospital that we have presented so far, and with that of most of the comparable accounts to which we have referred, is that it reflects an image presented by those who are themselves members of hospital teams. This is rather limited empirical evidence for, although such accounts are useful starting points, they convey (as we argue throughout this study) only a partial perspective. In order to explore more fully the practical impact of the ideal of an integrated service we shall therefore draw upon our field notes and upon interviews with relatives to examine two topics which we have selected for particular attention: the conduct of Tuesday meetings and the impact of the team of professionals upon relatives. At the end of the chapter we shall draw some conclusions about the success of the hospital more generally as an integrated service.

Team meetings

We have already noted the central role that the Tuesday meetings play in the work of the day hospital. The meetings are held in the treatment room at the day hospital, typically last about two hours (sometimes depending on the cases or other matters to be discussed but often depending upon the time that the consultant has available) and are attended by the consultant (who controls the meeting from the Chair), sister, senior enrolled nurse, social worker, nursing officer, secretary, community nurse, chiropodist, physiotherapist, occupational therapist, sisters or charge nurses from the three psychogeriatric wards in Park Hospital, and the Park Hospital administrator. Although attendance is, for the most part, very regular there are occasions when not all of these people are present.

The meetings are of a rather set format with clearly separate sections.

First, the administrator is asked if he has any topics for discussion. These might, for example, be the organization of transport or supply of materials. The items are generally brief and the administrator then leaves.

Second, the consultant asks the paramedical staff if they 'have anything'. Each in turn reports on what they see as any problems in dealing with the patients from the day hospital who have been referred to them for physiotherapy or other services. For the most part this is an exercise in reporting. Each paramedical has a 'turn' and when this section of the meeting is over the chiropodist and physiotherapist also leave.

Third, sisters or charge nurses report upon the progress of cases which have a connection with both the day hospital and Park Hospital. These may be in-patients attending the day hospital, day hospital patients admitted to a bed, short-term holiday admissions or whatever. Sometimes these staff use the occasion to discuss other in-patients with the consultant if they have been unable to gain access to him otherwise. Sometimes the consultant will use the occasion to allow ward and day hospital staff to press each other on points on which their interests diverge and on which he does not wish to be seen to adjudicate. (The use of the gardens by different groups of patients was one example.) At the end of this section of the meeting the ward staff also leave.

Fourth, new referrals are discussed. Since nearly all referrals come from GPs to the consultant, he reports the names of new cases and arranges for the social worker to visit them either before or after him. Thus psychiatric and social background reports are produced on most referrals. Other team members familiar with the case may comment at that stage.

Fifth, decisions are made on admissions and discharges. This process is complex and we have discussed it in detail in previous chapters. As we have shown, an understanding of these decisions must include, among other things, some description of the way in which professionals construe the problems of the elderly mentally infirm. The main points to note here are as follows. The major (and often only) contributors are the consultant, sister and social worker. It is they who have access to most information. If the consultant has a clear view, that view will generally prevail. If he does not, the discussion may flow. On occasions the sister and the social worker may exercise influence with a case carefully prepared in advance of the meeting.

Sixth, the sister reports on the progress of cases from the 'Kardex' nursing notes. She alone has access to this information in the meeting. The consultant may change a drug prescription or suggest treatment and the social worker may comment on the background factors. The occupational therapist may add information. Few major decisions are taken here although the groundwork is sometimes laid at this point for a subsequent decision on discharge.

Finally, if there is time any general policy or staff matters relating to the development of the day hospital are discussed, although this section of the meeting declined in importance as the hospital aged.

In order to give some impression of the character of these meetings, the following is an edited version of our field notes on one such occasion (the full note runs to some 8000 words):

> Dr McR [the consultant] announced the start of the meeting by asking Mr M [Park Hospital unit administrator] if he had any business. Mr M spoke about the O/T materials. He said he had made arrangements for the prices of the goods to be reduced. [He gave details.] Dr McR asked if there was anything else. Mr M said there wasn't, then Dr McR said that he had already mentioned the subject of [the availability of] beds, that he had written to Dr T about this. Mr M acknowledged that they had already discussed this. Mr M said the only matter he might mention was the subject of secretarial cover for the day hospital from his office. He had phoned Mrs D and it seemed that she was not likely to come back to work. He had suggested that in the circumstances it might be advisable for her to stay off. As her absence would be because of maternity leave the administration would only be able to make a temporary appointment to replace her. Dr McR asked if there was anything else and as Mr M was about to leave Mr B [nurse in charge of a Park Hospital ward] said that there is one thing he would like to mention. He had already discussed it with Mrs G [nursing officer] but wanted Mr M's advice. The matter concerned the census forms [which was fully discussed].
>
> Dr McR then turned to the chiropodist. She mentioned Mrs H and said that she could find nothing wrong with her feet. There had been some difficulty apparently with her walking, but she felt the problem stemmed from her knee and not her feet. The physio interjected at this point to say she also wanted to mention Mrs H. The problem was that Mrs H wore a very tight garter, so tight that it was restricting blood supply and had resulted in muscle atrophy. She mentioned some more technical points about this. The chiropodist mentioned that she had a huge varicose vein. Dr McR asked Nurse N [senior enrolled nurse standing in for sister, who was on leave] if there was any way of preventing her wearing these garters. Nurse N said that the patient was only attending the day hospital twice weekly and that made it difficult. Mrs X [social worker] suggested informing the relatives. During this exchange there were in fact several conversations going on regarding how they could possibly help in this situation and the fact that there were other patients who

also wore tight garters. Dr McR said that it was really quite serious, that the patient was demented and presumably she wouldn't understand why they wanted her to stop wearing the garter. He joked about a romper suit being the possible solution. Mrs G [nursing officer] entered the meeting and Mr B [charge nurse for Park Hospital] gave up his seat for her. The chiropodist said that the problem was as bad with Mrs H, that for these patients it had been a life-long habit and would be very difficult to change. Dr McR said that he would welcome any bright ideas.

Sister T [in charge of a Park Hospital ward] asked the physiotherapist if she had seen Mrs G and how she was doing. The physiotherapist said that she was walking, but would only do this whenever she wanted to. The social worker explained to Dr McR that this was the patient who comes to Park Hospital at weekends and who had remained there during the week because the son-in-law was ill and hadn't collected her. The chiropodist left the meeting and Mr B sat in her position.

The physiotherapist then mentioned Mrs F, the lady with a fractured patella who had difficulty getting on and off the bus. Nurse N said that they were now getting her off the bus backwards and that this seemed to be all right. Physio explained that she had suggested this and physiotherapy treatment. She left the meeting. Dr McR then turned to the business of the wards and asked if Mrs G was now in. Sister T [from the ward] said yes, but that she won't feed herself.

Dr McR asked the social worker what had happened in this case. Mrs X said that the son had been decanted [moved to another house for repairs to his own] a month ago but that he had since become ill and this was possibly a case of colic or infection. She had phoned the GP who said some tests had been clear but that the patient was to go back. The son-in-law had moved to live with his girl-friend and Mrs X didn't feel that they were going to get the patient back to him at the moment. Mrs G [nursing officer] commented, 'So she is taking up a bed'. Dr McR remarked that the situation wasn't very hopeful. He commented, 'She is in one of the spare beds that we tried not to use because of the redecoration [of the ward]'. There was some discussion on what beds had and had not been used. Dr McR thought that this patient might have to stay in this bed but at least it released half a bed, i.e. half of a shared bed, for other patients.

[After similar discussion of several other cases on the wards] the meeting was moved on by Dr McR running through minutes of the previous week; every point had been dealt with and he stopped at the subject of accepted patients. [Nurse N, in the absence of sister, reported briefly on the progress of each new patient.]

He then went on to Mrs T and asked if she was willing to attend. Mrs X [the social worker] thought she would have to be persuaded and compared her to [another case]. She thought attendance would be beneficial provided Dr McR also thought that attendance would help the patient 'to be lifted out of her depression'. This was agreed and times of attendance agreed.

[The nursing officer] asked if there was anything to talk about regarding short-stay beds. Dr McR said there was nothing desperate. She asked if they could be excused and she and the rest of the ward staff left.

[The community nurse] interrupted at this stage to say that while they were on the subject of sheltered housing he had another matter to bring up. Dr E had phoned him urgently about a Mrs N, a 91-year-old who was in [sheltered housing]. She is a problem during the day, and he wondered about getting her into the day hospital. Dr McR suggested that this should be referred to Mrs X in the usual way. The community nurse had interrupted rather apologetically and again apologized but he thought he would take the opportunity while they were on the subject of sheltered housing.

Dr McR said they would then go on to discuss referrals. He had a Mrs McB referred from [the town] – a 75-year-old in an old folks home. He had seen her yesterday – then decided it had been Friday. She was bright and cheerful and was a widow who had no children. She was approximately orientated for time, but she wanders. There are times when she thinks her husband is still alive and that he was ill and she has to go out to deal with this. The GP in his letter had said that the patient was demented, but Dr McR suggests that it is more a case of agitation. He read out an excerpt from the GP's letter, in which the GP said that he was under strong pressure from the matron of the home to have her removed. Dr McR said he would like to have Mrs X's views on this. He didn't necessarily see the patient coming here. He thought maybe it was a case for the waiting list. He thought that she should maybe be prescribed [medication] to take the steam out of her. She may just have to take her turn on the waiting list.

[Dr McR then went on to talk about several other referrals in a similar way, including] a Mr U of [town nearby], 'born 11.11.11.' He hadn't seen him yet but he wanted Mrs X to visit but not at the moment. He is a widower and lives with his two sisters-in-law. There seems to be some friction between them. He enjoys a whisky, he says, to a moderate extent. The sisters say he drinks to excess. According to the sisters his behaviour is bizarre. He gets up in the middle of the night and sets the fire. He can be aggressive and, according to the GP, they are saying that, 'something must be done'. The GP had to explain to them that Mr U was not as black as he was painted, but they had insisted on a visit by Dr McR. Reading between the lines Dr McR thought that the GP was suggesting that the relatives were trying it on. Dr McR said that was all they had. They certainly had plenty of referrals just now.

There was something he should have mentioned when [the administrator] was there, and that was an evening for the GPs. Dr McR would have to contact him about it. Mrs X thought the whole idea was very interesting. Dr McR said that it was difficult to know what numbers they would have. They would of course invite GPs in their catchment area. They would have to try and estimate the number and may have to limit them. It would be nice to have others but there would not be room to extend it much wider than this. The timing would either have to be quite soon or left till after the summer. Mrs X said that at least they had a start on it now. Dr McR said the main point of it was that the day hospital staff would be there for the GPs to talk to. It did of course mean that they were running the risk of getting more referrals. Mrs X thought it would be great to get through to them what the day hospital was all about. Dr McR said that he didn't think it would be necessary to have lengthy talks. Ten minutes from himself and Mrs X perhaps. He thought informality was best.

[After some further discussion about GPs there followed a lengthy interruption by the community nurse about possible day-hospital attendance by two patients being considered for discharge from in-patient care in the area psychiatric hospital.]

Nurse N said there was also Mrs C whose relatives say she is hallucinating. She is not on any medication. She wondered about her being put on [medication]. The relatives are requesting a holiday bed. Mrs X went out of the meeting to get dates. Nurse N and Mrs X had had an an interchange before this. I think it was concerning the following patient rather than this one.

Nurse N went on to say that Mrs D's sister was in a very bad state and that if something was not done soon then it would be necessary to find two beds. The sister's weight was down to five stones. She was requesting a holiday admission for Mrs D. Dr McR said that he was a bit concerned that if they take patients on at the day hospital and don't have any beds that he can use, then perhaps the patients don't get their share of beds [at another psychiatric hospital]. The community nurse said he thought they did all right, that problems come to light more readily in this situation. Nurse N said that this was a very difficult patient and described the problems as, 'She is very noisy and is quite a strain on the staff in the day hospital' and she felt it would be very difficult to live with her.

Nurse N then went on to Mrs I. Her daughters were having a terrible time. She is defecating all over the place and the daughters have young children which makes it even more difficult. She really requires a long-term bed. Mrs X referred back to the previous evening's relatives' meeting. The district nurse [who had been at the meeting as a speaker] had been interested in this case and had suggested going to give the patient an enema. Nurse N said otherwise there were no other problems with this patient. Mrs X said the daughters want to cope but are just not the type to be able to. Nurse N said they both worked. Someone then told a story about a patient in an old folks' home who hadn't been to the toilet for about two months and was then incontinent and there was a lot of joking about this. They also joked that I was not to write this down.

Dr McR asked Mrs X if she had anything. She presumed Mrs N was not going home and wondered if she could give up the house as it required a month's notice. Dr McR confirmed that there was no chance if her living alone and that she could go ahead with this. [There was then further case discussion with the community nurse.]

After this, discussion broke up and everyone left. Both [the social worker] and [the community nurse] were commenting about how useful the informal discussions were in facilitating good staff relationships. Mrs X said that she felt that perhaps Dr McR did not get much opportunity to talk to staff and that he would very much like to be part of the team, but this was not so easy to do in practice because of the time commitments.

On the basis of these and similar data, and with the topic of this chapter in mind, we observe that the Tuesday meeting functions as a key element in the organization of services by a team of professionals in the following way:

(1) The paramedical staff are limited in their influence within a clearly confined organizational space. The chiropodist, for example, speaks only about the chiropody aspects of patient care and then only when asked to do so. When the topic of chiropody is over, she leaves. In practice, here, teamwork means specialization and the ready provision of a range of professional services to which patients can be referred by sister and the consultant in charge.
(2) The meeting is a clear expression of the interdependent relationship that exists between sister and the consultant. While the consultant is clearly dependent upon her for much information, the occasion also serves as a public display of the authority which sister exercises with consultant support. Thus the medical hierarchies of control are reinforced rather than undermined on these occasions.
(3) The meeting also institutionalizes and confines organizationally (and thus renders manageable) the interface between social work and psychiatric services and specialisms. The day hospital has not really solved the problem of providing a co-ordinated social work/psychiatric service to patients. It has incorporated an element of social work into the medical system of care and in support of medical practice. But this has been achieved at the cost of considerably weakening the links between this element of social work and the rest of the social work department. The social worker *assists* the psychiatrist. The consultant's public espousal of the social worker's worth brings her considerable prestige but allows

her to influence the consultant only minimally. Although the social worker sees herself as quite successful in having introduced a 'social perspective' into the hospital, the major outcome is that the consultant gains a social work service – in particular a route to local authority domiciliary and residential care.
(4) Thus generally the meeting reasserts rather than revolutionizes traditional hospital patterns of work and divisions of labour. Although some overlap occurs between some staff roles (for example, between social work and the community nurse or between nursing and occupational therapy) this is marginal and not threatening to core skills which are, if anything, consolidated. Therefore the structure of the team which is designed to facilitate co-ordination, itself generates the need for co-ordinating machinery because it institutionalizes a highly specialized division of labour.
(5) Particularly importantly, however, the holding of this meeting and the occurrence of 'rituals' of consultation and decision-making, serve to foster an image of team activity and allow staff of all grades and specialities to value this as an end in itself. Although much that happens at this meeting could actually be accomplished without the meeting, its importance lies in the fact that it maintains the myth of team work, co-ordinated services and thus 'success'.
(6) The meeting bolsters the consultant's role and power position in several ways. Within the meeting he balances the interests of various staff groups against each other – especially ward and day-hospital staff. He moves between making and declining to make decisions.
(7) The meeting serves as a mechanism for protecting staff against relatives' demands. Relatives have an interest in gaining information about their patients and in bombarding staff with demands for admission or discharge. The notion of some corporate responsibility allows staff on occasions to escape what they may feel to be individual harassment by resort to the team and by avowing lack of power to the relatives. Individual relations seeking to pressurize the hospital may find it difficult to isolate a precise target against which to direct their efforts.

Overall it is difficult to avoid the conclusion that much of the decision-making within the meeting is apparent rather than real, that the meeting reinforces traditional power and hierarchial relations and diverts attention from the lack of innovation by rituals held up *ipso facto* as beneficial. These maintain the image of successful integrated service.

The impact on relatives

The attempt to provide a range of integrated services by a team of professionals at the day hospital is not generally apparent to relatives. They do not experience co-ordinated provision. Relatives typically experience a fragmented and disparate system of services. This is because the team approach at the day hospital does not effectively extend co-ordination to the main health and social-work services received by the patients and their carers.

There is considerable variation in the circumstances in which patients come to attend the day hospital. In most instances the first contact is with the patient's

GP and it is through their GP that most cases are referred to the day hospital. Many relatives, however, do not understand the process of referral and admission. In particular they do not understand the relationship between the assessment visits by the consultant and the social worker, and the impact that these visits may have on the decision to admit. The pathway to the day hospital is often further complicated for relatives by the fact that GPs themselves frequently have no clear picture of the workings of the day hospital or the system of allocation of places. Relatives thus often experience delay before referral is initiated by the GP and receive mixed messages about the extent of help that they are likely to receive. The team approach at the day hospital has done little to smooth this pathway and provide an experience of co-ordinated services for relatives en route to the institution.

The disjunction in perception between relatives and staff continues after patient admission. For example, we have already pointed to the way in which in-patient beds are used in conjunction with day hospital places. However, although the practice has increased the number and frequency of short-term relief admissions, relatives experience the process as haphazard and not necessarily in keeping with their needs.

The following case illustrates these points. Mr and Mrs N approached their GP early in the year to request the short-term admission of their patient in order to take two weeks' holiday in July. Although the relatives were experiencing a great deal of difficulty, their GP said that little could be done for the patient and did not make a referral to the day hospital. In our interview with her, Mrs N explained the outcome of her approach to the GP:

> MRS N: 'Well the doctor got in touch with somebody and it was a health visitor that came first and then another social worker.'
> MR N: '... and the doctor [another doctor] came tae.'
> MRS N: 'Aye, a Dr P came to see about getting him into a home.'
> INTERVIEWER: 'All these people were about getting a holiday break?'
> MRS N: 'Aye, and the first social worker that came – I was really sick disgusted with him because he was asking all the questions which we had answered about five times before and he says, "I have only twelve vacancies for the Fair Holidays and I have allocated seven of them this morning." I mean it was the first time we had tried ...'

Meantime the patient was referred and admitted to the day hospital. In March the social worker there visited the family and said that in her view, the patient was not suitable for a social work department residential home. She would try to have him admitted to an in-patient bed in Park Hospital for the holiday period. Some months before the period for which they had requested a holiday admission the relatives were offered in-patient accommodation for two weeks. The relatives said that this admission had come as a surprise to them and had not been at their request, although the relief was very welcome. Mrs N explained that the social worker had suggested it. The social worker said that the consultant had mentioned the availability of a bed at one of their conferences, and she had asked if this patient could have it. However the day hospital was not able to provide a bed during the relatives' annual holiday period and, despite the social worker's earlier comments about the patient's unsuitability for local authority residential accommodation, an area-based social worker proceeded with what proved to be an unsuccessful attempt to obtain the holiday admission in social work department accommodation.

Although staff claim that the day hospital has increased the likelihood of this type of case obtaining short-term admission, the social worker and the consultant had not managed effectively to mesh resource allocation with family needs. This example also illustrates the way in which the day hospital team does little to increase overall co-operation between the health services and the social work department.

Patients who are attending the day hospital are likely to be receiving a battery of other services from the social work department. Also they still require the services of a GP. To some extent the day hospital does effectively collaborate with these other services. For example, home-help visits are timed to enable the home help to ensure that the patient is ready when the day hospital transport arrives. GPs are routinely informed by the day hospital of significant medical developments with the patient and they issue prescriptions on the recommendation of the day hospital doctors. However, there are quite severe limits to this kind of co-ordination between the day hospital team and external services. GPs are not routinely provided with comprehensive details about the treatment and progress of patients. For example, they do not receive any information about the occupational therapist's work with patients. Neither can social work department domiciliary services always be provided to cover the periods when the patient is not attending the day hospital.

Relatives also experience the limited effectiveness of the team approach at the point of discharge. One relative, for example, complained:

> ... The way the system is going just now everybody wants something for nothing, everybody is all that busy keeping themselves out of trouble. One department does not know what the other department is doing. Its true. When she was in the care of the day centre down there the nurses [i.e. the district nurses] would have nothing to do with her ... of course it is not their problem. That problem is down at [the day hospital]. And then when [the day hospital] was finished with her they palmed her on to the district nurse and now the health visitor has nothing more to do with her. The social worker has nothing else to do with her.

We have already mentioned the relatives' group and in Chapter 10 we shall consider fully its functions within the system of the hospital. But for the purposes of the present discussion it is relevant to highlight one or two points for this also is a context in which we might expect relatives to experience the benefits of a team approach.

The group of staff concerned with organizing the meetings of the relatives is significant. The social worker is the central figure. Sister is active. The senior enrolled nurse, and sometimes the secretary and occupational therapist, attend. The consultant attends only very rarely as a 'special guest speaker'. In the history of the group it is also significant that, at least initially, its activities met with some resistance from nursing officers and administrators. They saw the hospital as being concerned with providing medical services to patients and were clearly dubious about the place of this 'social activity' within the Health Service. More to the point, they were very wary about the degree of influence and automony that the social worker was apparently exercising and made several, largely unsuccessful, attempts to 'supervise' nursing staff involved in the group by 'dropping in' from time to time. The issue was particularly delicate since nursing staff do not wear uniform at the meetings and are not paid overtime for that evening's 'work'.

In the light of these points, and of the more detailed account that we give elsewhere, observation of the relatives' meetings suggested that it functions in the following way as part of the organization and provision of a range of services by a group of professional staff.

First, as we have noted, staff in the meeting use the 'team' to avoid 'relative pressure'.

Second, the meetings provide an arena in which the social worker can very visibly exercise considerable influence and control over hospital services. We have already described how this is important as a part of the 'social exchange' between social worker and medical staff. However just as relatives are substantially confined here (we develop this argument fully in Chapter 10) so too the influence of the social worker in the team is considerably less outside the relatives' group and does not seriously impinge on the traditional areas of medical concern.

Third, as in staff meetings, staff in relatives' meetings tend to confine their comments to their own area of professional expertise. The contributions of the occupational therapist, sister and social worker, in particular, are very much based upon a 'division of labour' rather than a 'pooling of resources'.

Fourth, a rather select group of staff attend these meetings. Apart from the notable absence of the consultant, there is no representation of that group of staff which actually has day-to-day contact with many relatives – the nursing auxiliaries (who staff the bus run, amongst other duties). The staff involved in these meetings are those who tend to have the closest links with each other anyway. The absence, too, of the medical officer, means that from the relatives' perspective many of their concerns about the co-ordination of services remain unanswered.

Finally, these meetings do not fulfil the task of helping relatives with problems of co-ordintion between day hospital and other services for the elderly mentally confused. At relatives' meetings the crucial problems of relating hospital and GP services appear as intractable as ever.

Conclusion

We began this chapter by reviewing the literature on some comparable day hospitals for the elderly mentally infirm. This describes the range of psychiatric, medical, social work and associated services commonly provided in psychogeriatric day hospitals and the way in which staff providing these services work together. Typically team work is described as an important feature, together with the existence of a wide range of services, and an *esprit de corps* amongst staff. In spite of some role ambiguity and uncertainty about traditional hierarchies of control, services of a high order are generally adjudged to be the result.

Although the account given by staff of the day hospital that we have studied largely conforms to this description, our field notes on observations and interviews with relatives are less sanguine about the success of the institution in providing an integrated service. We have concentrated in this chapter upon the conduct of staff meetings and upon the impact of the 'integrated' service on relatives – in the relatives' group and more widely.

To generalize from these various materials, the attempt to provide a range of psychogeriatric and related services through a team of professional staff within the day hospital has the following consequences. The division of labour within the team tends to confirm the boundaries between existing specialisms. Social-work services are incorporated into the work of the hospital but without disturbing the usual professional hierarchies of medical practice. The day hospital has not really solved the problem of providing a co-ordinated social work and psychiatric service to patients since, even when the services provided within the hospital are effectively co-ordinated, crucial issues remain concerning the co-ordination of hospital services with those provided by outside agencies. Park Hospital staff are not viewed as full team members. Much service provision is in practice quite highly segmented. The major problem of co-ordinating day hospital services with those provided from general practice has not been significantly affected. The most significant development in integrated resource use – the use of in-patient beds in Park Hospital in close conjunction with day hospital places – has taken place outside of the day hospital team.

From the point of view of relatives, provision of integrated services by a team of professionals does not necessarily result in a more coherent picture of services or in the experience of co-ordinated service provision from the day hospital. There is a discrepancy between staff views of integrated provision and relatives' experience of a fragmented and disparate system of services. This is because the team approach at the day hospital does not effectively extend co-ordination to the main health and social work services received from other sources by patients and their relatives. Relatives frequently experience the processes of access to, receipt of and discharge from the services of the day hospital as haphazard and not necessarily fitting in with their needs. The central point is that patients attending the day hospital are likely to be receiving a battery of other services, and although the day hospital collaborates effectively with some of these services relatives see little being done to minimize the major problems of co-ordination between services which arise for them at crucial points in the patient's career through the day hospital.

In the next chapter we turn specifically to this issue of the relationship between the day hospital and related services.

CHAPTER EIGHT

Success as Impact on Related Services

Introduction

Although the research reported in this book is primarily a case study of one day hospital, it is important to remember that this hospital is a part of a wider system of care for the elderly mentally infirm in the area.

This feature of the hospital is of some importance to its staff and our respondents explained forcefully to us that one of the major ways in which the work of the hospital should be evaluated lies in assessing its contribution to other services. It is claimed, for example, that the day hospital relieves pressure on other services by helping to reduce demand where it is excessive. It is also felt that the day hospital is a genuine part of an overall system of care through interaction between staff and through the cross-referral of patients at admission and discharge. There is the strong view that through these activities the day hospital should improve the quality and efficacy of service provision in the system as a whole. These points were made in relation to a number of individual services with which the day hospital has some kind of contact, either through links between staff or through the system of patient flow within the overall structure of care for the elderly mentally infirm. The essential argument is that if the day hospital allows other professional groups to perform their duties more effectively, then this is an important indirect benefit stemming from the establishment of the hospital.

Although we have repeatedly mentioned these links between the day hospital and other institutions in our discussions of patient flow, clinical cure and an integrated service, we have some difficulty in discussing the hospital in terms of this criterion since a study which would effectively assess it in this way would have been designed from the start quite differently from this piece of research. We conducted a case study of the institution from the 'inside out'. This has a number of very important advantages and we have tried to capitalize upon them in presenting our data. In particular we have been able to explore some subjects in considerable depth. But the approach does have some disadvantages as well. We are not, and never expected to be, in a position to assess the impact of the day hospital upon the overall system of care. Such a study would have to be a much larger one and would focus on a set of interrelated institutions caring for the elderly, rather than principally upon a single organization (see Hunter and Cantley 1984). Undoubtedly there are arguments in favour of evaluative research taking a system perspective (although we would argue for the advantages of it following the pluralistic approach adopted in this research). Clearly a perfect set of research results would embody both detailed case studies and an overview of the system as a whole. The problem is that for most practical purposes such a research exercise would be extremely difficult to mount, expensive, time consuming and very unwieldy.

Nevertheless, having made this qualification, some of our material is not unrelated to issues of the relationships which the day hospital has to other services and although we cannot answer the question, 'What is the impact of the day hospital upon the overall system of care?' we can describe the contribution which staff think that the hospital is making. We can also examine our research materials to see whether or not the data are consistent with the perspectives which staff have on the role of the hospital in this respect.

This chapter therefore deals in turn with the impact that the day hospital has on a number of services: general practice, field and residential social work, the rest of the psychiatric system, Park Hospital, the geriatric services, and finally domiciliary services. Our general conclusion is that relationships between the day hospital and related services vary considerably. Our data are in some instances consistent with the view that the hospital is contributing to the effectiveness of these services. In other instances we have some reservations.

General practice

The GP service is the first and most obvious point at which the day hospital may contribute to the work of another service. Respondents suggested that the day hospital simply has more time than GPs to care for elderly patients. Certainly we have already suggested that the medical officer is, in effect, relieving GPs of some of their workload.

> [GPs] are in a busy practice. How much time can you devote, an elderly person comes and says, 'Doctor' ... it will take a long time, it will be much longer than even now to assess that person; he cannot cope with it so he is passing it to us and we have got an expert psychiatrist, we've got the person under surveillance so to speak ...
>
> (*A nursing administrator*)

> We offer the community an almost immediate service in that we offer relief for – and I am talking about GPs, and that doesn't always happen in other places ... that you get immediate relief and when I talk about immediate relief it can be immediate ... now that relieves the doctor, because it takes the pressure off him.

It relieves the pressure from the relatives getting on to him about something getting done.

(*A social worker*)

And as a nursing sister explained:

We certainly relieve the GP in a lot of cases where he had hysterical, hypochondrical patients at him all the time, that's taken away because, they feel, we seem to take over as long as we've got - someone's listening to them, someone dealing with their problems, we take over so we relieve a lot in the community and a lot of the services that are in the community.

Of course, as we have already explained, the way in which we would like to be able to assess these claims is to draw, amongst other materials, on data reporting GPs' perceptions of the day hospital. For reasons which we have also explained, data of this kind are not available within this study. Nevertheless we do have data which allow us to make *some* comments on the way in which day hospital services may be affecting the work of GPs. Furthermore, a good deal of material relevant to this point has already been presented in our discussions of the day hospital's attempt to provide an active therapeutic regime and also in our discussion of the hospital's attempt to provide an integrated and interlinked set of services through a team of professional workers. The material on the GPs' perspective on issues of patient flow is relevant too. The discussion that follows will therefore present some new data but will also recall these other materials.

As we have documented, a major proportion of referrals to the day hospital come from GPs, only a small proportion coming either from psychiatrists or from geriatricians or other medical practitioners. It may be the case that GPs are referring on some cases which have been referred to them by non-medical professionals, although there is little evidence in our sample from GP referral letters that this is so. Our strong impression is that the vast majority of GP referrals are already cases on the GP's list and are cases with which the GP has been very actively concerned.

We cannot tell what proportion of the GP's overall active workload such cases represent but we can tell from the ways in which these cases are described in GP referral letters that in many cases they are a serious concern to GPs who feel that they are no longer able to offer the intense attention that they consider the cases require. The flavour of such referrals is contained in the following note taken from the file of one patient:

Dr C requests a domiciliary visit on this old man. He lives with his elderly wife who looks after him. He is the usual arteriosclerotic condition - has been seen by Dr T, the geriatrician consultant at [a local hospital] and his name is on the geriatric waiting list. However there is a much greater deterioration in his mental condition since February. He is attacking his old wife and elderly sister-in-law, sits and masturbates for hours, strips off his clothes and goes out in the street and is very threatening.

The following is a further example. This is described in a letter from the GP:

This woman shows the classical signs and symptoms of senile dementia due to cerebral arteriosclerosis. She lives alone and is vehemently independent, and over the last twelve months has been becoming increasingly more disoriented in time and place and is now wandering around [the town] at all hours of the day and night. She has had two episodes of electrical fires due to leaving appliances on for long periods. Luckily she has extremely good neighbours, and her niece and these neighbours have taken the brunt of the work ... I would be grateful if you would see her and if you would telephone or contact her niece, then she could try and keep the old lady at home.

Without the services of the day hospital such problems would continue to be primarily the responsibility of GPs. In this case the day hospital can justifiably claim to be offering 'relief'.

In discussions of referrals to the day hospital at the Tuesday meetings, the views of the referring practitioners are certainly of considerable significance, especially if the GP reports that the patient is proving particularly troublesome. We have already presented one extract from a Tuesday meeting which described the 'trouble' that was caused to a GP by two patients (see Chapter 6, pp. 79–82). In another case our field notes record the way in which the GP's views had been important in deciding that a case should be a psychogeriatric rather than a geriatric referral.

[The consultant] now mentioned Mrs McD .. he had phoned the GP about her physical state to suggest that this be passed to Dr F [the geriatrician]. The GP had been reluctant to do this. Dr F would not want this case because of its psychiatric components. It was difficult to know which way to jump and he gave some examples of this. [The consultant] however agreed that something must be done in this case...

However, we would not want to imply that the GPs' views go totally unquestioned and referers who paint too gloomy a picture of their case may well lose the sympathy of the hospital, as the following case shows. Our field notes record:

[The consultant] said there was one possible case, Mr S. Social worker said she had also seen him. [The consultant] said that this man was a 59-year-old man from [a nearby town]. He was very unsteady on his feet and his movements were jerky ... He had also been depressed. [The consultant] had got him into [a psychiatric hospital] in the past and he had improved then ... since then he has had another couple of spells in [the psychiatric hospital] ... [The consultant] said that this man had been home for the past year. The GP had requested a domiciliary visit as he had deteriorated and was staying in bed all day etc. [The consultant] made an evening visit and the patient had himself opened the door. There was general amusement about this. [The consultant] had found him to be in the same position as before ... [In the end the meeting concluded that] day care was a misuse of facilities in this case as Mr S was very fit and would go on for years.

Also, apart from the fact that not all of their referrals are accepted, there are other limitations on the service which the day hospital offers to general practitioners in respect of their difficult patients.

GPs are by no means fully relieved of responsibility for patients attending the day hospital. The GP remains responsible for general medical treatment for any problems which arise with the patient outside the immediate period of day hospital attendance. The GP is, too, responsible for the continued prescription of medicines for day hospital patients. There was the case, for example, in which a patient who was bitten by a dog had to attend the GP to obtain a tetanus injection even though the patient was attending the day hospital (indeed, attendance at the day hospital meant that it was rather difficult to arrange a suitable appointment with the GP). This continuing responsibility of the GP is confirmed by the responses we received from relatives when we interviewed them. For the most part, relatives continue to view the patient's GP as the primary source of medical care for the patient. The day hospital is an additional facility but not a substitute for the GP, and the battery of services which the hospital offers is not seen as a substitute for primary medical care. Although the medical officer at the day hospital does inform the GP of any medical problems which he identifies and treats, there is no regular procedure for conveying to GPs a general picture of the course of the patient's improvement or deterioration. At discharge the GP is informed by the hospital of the fact of discharge and the reasons for that decision but, contrary to decision-making at admission, GPs' views do not play any significant part in the decision to terminate day hospital treatment.

In certain respects, the day hospital creates some problems for GPs. The day hospital seeks a rapid throughput of patients and is, as we have discussed, concerned to keep patients in 'the community'. Such patients remain the responsibility of 'community services' of which the GP service is one. The practice of intermittent readmissions in particular is likely to generate difficulties for GPs. Staff in the day hospital are conscious of this point. It was made by one of our respondents, a senior nurse:

> GPs in the area [are concerned] for their own job. They want the patient removed from the community and put into a ward, because that takes the onus off of them and they are safe and secure in a hospital ward and you were always going to come up against the problems of that because you are going to try the opposite and reverse it and keep the patient in their own home and the GPs wouldn't like that. We always knew that and it would put a stress on every service in the community . . .

Indeed, if the initiative of a day hospital has entailed the use of health authority resources for day care rather than for making provision for additional in-patient beds, and if many GPs are really seeking a permanent in-patient bed for the patients which they refer to the day hospital, then it could be said that the day hospital is creating problems for GPs. For by diverting resources from those forms of provision which GPs are really seeking, the day hospital is delaying their being relieved completely of responsibility for some of their most difficult patients.

Social work

A second service to which the day hospital relates is social work. As we have explained, the social work services within the day hospital are provided by a member of the local authority social work department who works almost exclusively in the day hospital but who also provides a more limited service to Park Hospital. Although the social worker is a member of a hospital-based team with a senior social worker in a nearby general hospital, the boundaries of the catchment area of the day hospital are not coterminous with the social work department boundaries so that the social worker must liaise with a large number of different social work offices in organizing services for day hospital patients.

There is a range of social work department provisions which involve patients; home-help services, meals on wheels, residential accommodation, day care, social casework and short-term holiday accommodation. We consider field and residential social work services in this section and deal with social work department domiciliary services along with Health Services domiciliary services below.

In spite of the fact that there is a good deal of contact between the day hospital and social workers in the local authority social work department, the majority of staff in the day hospital did not mention this as an area in which the day hospital is contributing to any significant extent. Only the social worker was an exception. She spoke about her involvement in mediating between the day hospital and the social work department over the transfer of patients and other matters. Since the social worker is the only member of the day hospital staff who has any extensive contact with other social workers, it is perhaps not surprising that the day hospital staff have little conception of the effect of the day hospital in this respect.

In the last chapter we dealt quite fully with the part that the day hospital social worker plays in co-ordinating health and social work services. Here, however, one or two further comments are in order. We can make some assessment of the degree to which day hospital services alleviate the difficulties which the local authority social work department might otherwise have in dealing with difficult clients.

Contact between the day hospital and the social work department arises in a number of contexts. First there are those cases which are effectively referred to the day hospital by social workers (although, of course, the referral would come via a GP). We saw little evidence either in the patient files or in the material that we collected at Tuesday meetings, to suggest that field social workers are in practice referring any significant number of cases to the day hospital. Our strong impression is that patients who are proving troublesome while in contact with a *field* social worker are likely also to be in contact with their GP, who will refer them to the day hospital direct (although, as we have pointed out, our data are not strong in making this kind of assessment). However we have clear evidence that a significant proportion of the cases admitted to the day hospital are referred, in effect, by those in charge of local authority or voluntary residential accommodation where the patient is proving difficult. Of our sample of forty-five admissions, four were in local authority *residential* accommodation of some kind at the time of first attending the day hospital. A further case was in a home run by a voluntary organization. The following social background report describes one such case:

> Mrs N is a 92-year-old widow who lives in sheltered housing in a linked residential unit. She is taken from her home daily into the residential part of the [residential] home. She apparently can be quite aggressive and extremely noisy at times. She proclaims to be the Queen of Sheba and quite often becomes high-handed and

> rough with other residents. Because of this there is much pressure being put on the matron of the home to have Mrs N removed from the unit. In order to share some of this burden I would recommend that day care be offered two days a week meantime.

Notes on file give some indication of the disruptive behaviour of two further patients who were admitted to the day hospital while in a residential home:

> Patient very confused. Causing a lot of trouble, wandering outside. Hallucinations – over dead husband. Can't sleep. Very depressed.
>
> This old man suffers from senile dementia. He keeps on pushing the other men out of their beds and is generally causing havoc. He wanders from the home and is then brought back by the police.

We are unable to present a view of the situation from the perspective of social workers responsible for residential accommodation but it seems most likely that the removal of disruptive patients from a residential home to day-hospital accommodation for at least some period each week would be welcomed.

However there are two sides to the equation, for the day hospital also makes some demands upon the social work department for residential accommodation and other services. Some patients are discharged from the day hospital to residential or day care provided by the social work department. There are, too, occasions on which the day hospital seeks short-term provision of residential accommodation from the social work department for patients whose relatives are going on holiday or need a short break for some other reason. But as we have shown in Chapter 5, the numbers involved here are not large. In our sample of admitted cases only two went to local authority day care on discharge, and only one case in our sample was admitted to short-term local authority accommodation to provide 'holiday relief' for relatives (although this may be something of an underestimate since this particular detail is not always clearly recorded in the case file if the patient was not at the same time discharged from the day hospital).

This does not mean that the day hospital does not perform a substantial amount of work which can legitimately be described as providing a social-work service. It may well be regarded as relieving the social work department of the care of some clients who would otherwise necessarily be its concern. However, there are two points to be emphasized in the context of the present discussion. The first is that the social worker is an employee of the social work department but with a workload generated almost entirely from within the hospital. The major activities of the social worker – preparing background reports, dealing with home emergencies of patients attending the hospital, organizing the relatives' group, negotiating with social work authorities in connection with patient discharge – are activities geared to the organization and concerns of the hospital. In that sense the social worker at the day hospital is not a resource which other social workers within the social work department can employ. Rather, he or she is a social work resource for the consultant psychiatrist and others within the system of medical care. The social work activity which takes place as a result of the establishment of the day hospital represents no net increase in social work resources in this field of care but rather a redistribution of resources – effectively, the movement of one social work post from the social work department to the Health Service.

The second point to note is that those cases which are in contact with the social worker in the day hospital are not handled totally by that social worker. In that sense the social worker does not hold a 'case load' as a member, for example, of an area team. Rather the social worker is concerned only with those aspects of the case which have a bearing upon the patient's attendance at the day hospital. It is therefore necessary for a field social worker to remain in contact with a case if, for example, that case was known to the social work department before admission to the day hospital.

Psychiatry

A further area of interservice contact is that between the day hospital and the wider psychiatric system of which it is a part. Indeed, as we have already described, one of the main rationales for the establishment of the day hospital was that it should ease the existing pressure of work on an overburdened psychiatric service.

In assessing the success of the day hospital in terms of its impact upon other psychiatric services, one relevant issue is thus whether or not the hospital has provided consultants with an additional resource when dealing with psychiatric referrals. One administrator commented upon the day hospital's performance:

> INTERVIEWER: 'In a general way, how would you describe the service that the day hospital is offering?'
> ADMINISTRATOR: 'I think it's given the consultants, who are placed in a very difficult position when they're called to see a patient who is in need of treatment and – relatives who are in need of a break – an opportunity other than offering them a full-time residence in a psychiatric hospital, with all the stigma that that still means to many people, the opportunity of great support and some help to their relatives at the same time on a day basis, not a psychiatric hospital but to a day hospital, and I think its *most helpful* for the consultant to be able to go in and say, "I can offer you something positively".'
> INTERVIEWER: 'So its offering an additional resource and avenue . . .?'
> ADMINISTRATOR: 'Exactly. And one that – that's always available and perhaps quickly because of the policy [on patient flow] that we've got. It maintains him always in this position where he has got something to offer, and he is not finding himself in a position where he can do nothing, nothing either for the patient, nothing for the relative [As if to say] 'I have nothing to offer, and I have not even a suggestion to make.'

And it is is not only the consultant psychiatrist who benefits from the availability of day-hospital places. A community psychiatric nurse involved with psychogeriatric cases commented that '. . . as far as I was concerned on a personal basis, it gave me a second avenue for dealing with psychogeriatrics from the community.'

As well as providing additional facilities, one of the original hopes for the day hospital was that it should relieve the demand for in-patient beds. A psychiatrist assessed its impact in this respect as follows:

INTERVIEWER: 'In terms of its original objective of relieving pressure on beds, do you think that has contributed much really?'

CONSULTANT: 'Yes. Its relieved pressure on psychiatrists I think! [Laughs]. I don't know whether it has made any impact on the waitintg list or not – eh – because – hm – the waiting list is probably tending to increase anyway. I suspect that if we – hm – looked at the male psychogeriatric patients, I think we might see a reduction in certainly of urgent cases, because we've taken quite a lot of male patients, I think, either on a long-term or short-term, but I don't think we'd see any different in the female psychogeriatric waiting list and that of course is because the demand is so high, so that there's no question of us being able to say because the day hospital is here therefore we can take down some of the beds, we're a long, long way from that – so anybody who's hoping to see that kind of effect I think will be disappointed, on the female side anyway.'

So often, as this quotation shows, the question of whether or not the day hospital has contributed to the rest of the psychiatric sector comes back to the issue of whether or not it has successfully increased the flow of patients through parts of the system which were previously blocked. We discussed this topic very fully in Chapter 5, on patient flow, and our conclusions here are the same. The day hospital *may* be delaying the admission of some patients to in-patient beds (we have argued that this is doubtful) but there is little evidence to suggest that it is diverting patients from this demand. Patients are moved in and out of the day hospital itself and in this respect the psychiatrist's problems are eased by his being provided with an additional source of help for the excessive number of cases which are referred to him.

And here, perhaps, is an important key to understanding the impact which the day hospital is having on other services. Although we are not in a position to assess this impact from the perspective of professionals providing these services, we *are* in a position to say something about the relative effort which groups within the hospital make in shaping their contribution. The important point is that, in some areas, influential groups within the day hospital actually have a vested interest in maintaining the operation of the day hospital as a relatively self-contained system and in *not* developing links with other services, even where such potential exists. We have already shown that, in contact with GPs and social workers, the service offered by the hospital is quite specifically limited. In the case of the day hospital's relations with other parts of the psychiatric sector, however, it is certainly in the psychiatrist's interests to ease the problems of patient flow because the consultant psychiatrist is himself, in another role, a part of that wider psychiatric system. Thus the general pluralistic model which we have advanced, and which seeks to explain much of what happens in the day hospital in terms of the vested interests of its numerous groups, has relevance in this context also.

Park Hospital

We have described the relationship between the day hospital and Park Hospital. In Chapter 5 we also dealt with the movement of patients between the two institutions and considered the differing interests of day hospital and Park

Hospital staff. Day hospital staff, however, do not consider that their impact should be confined to increasing patient turnover in the previously static in-patient wards. (And in any case, as we showed, they are not very successful on that count.) A consultant explained what he saw as the other advantages to Park Hospital of having the day hospital in such close proximity:

> CONSULTANT: 'You know people say, "Oh! gosh! Park!" and they don't often put it on the same footing as [the general hospital] but for all that it does a tremendous amount of work. Now – eh – I have a feeling that the siting of the day hospital here has done something for Park, I may be wrong about that, but I think it has brought more attention on Park . . .'
> INTERVIEWER: 'From the medical . . . ?'
> CONSULTANT: 'From – eh – from the administrative, from the district and from the areas, Park must have been mentioned more often – eh – now I'm not saying – I don't know whether at the same time it may have brought a certain amount of y'know there's always certain rivalries and so on in any institution, I don't know whether it has promoted any of these feelings, but I would think on the whole it has been good for the hospital and I don't know, but I think – hm – possibly there may have been a doubt about Park's future, there always is about an old hospital and – eh – this must surely have done something to reassure people that the hospital has a future, but I'm really sort of guessing here, it's just a funny sort of feeling that – eh – in some way, [the day hospital] being here has – eh – has helped Park.'

Park Hospital staff also derive some benefit from the proximity of the day hospital. By attending the day hospital's weekly Tuesday meetings they gain increased access to the consultant. For the staff of Park Hospital there are also some spin-off effects of some day hospital practices. For example, background information which the social worker obtains on the admission of a patient to the day hospital can later prove to be useful to Park Hospital staff when the patient is admitted long-term. A nurse explained:

> . . . the information one sometimes would get, when a patient is admitted to – as a long-stay patient for example, is in most cases very sketchy – background-wise. Its once the patient is in, that you've to try in going from various sources for information about the patient, it can sometimes take years, you then find out, 'Oh! so-and-so – oh! He has a relative', y'know, you've thought this man may be hasn't any next of kin at all, whereas with, hm – the patients at the day hospital, and possibly because of the social worker going and actually making a point of getting this information approaching other bodies who may – other parties who may have this information from this, the district nurse or the GP or whoever, – hm – we've got as full a picture as it's possible to get about the patient, and I think this is necessary and this helps in the long run when a patient is admitted to a long-stay ward.

Geriatric services

The problems of limited recources in the provision of geriatric services and the interest of the geriatrician were both clearly influential in the planning of the day hospital. There was a definite expectation that the day hospital would provide assistance to geriatrics as well as to psychiatry. In the mind of the planners the problems of the two sectors were closely interrelated. One administrator explained:

> Well, the main goals of the day hospital I think we saw – somewhat pragmatically perhaps, being an answer to this – eh – *enormous* problem of how we were going to treat the elderly. For Dr H, our consultant geriatrician, had made it quite clear that as well as this problem I have described of elderly patients in [the psychiatric hospital] being treated in a less than adequate setting, equally he argued that he in the geriatric side had a considerable number of patients who were *very* confused, who were getting to be dementia patients, who were being looked after in an acute sort of setting, you know an *acute* geriatric setting, and that he neither had the resources nor the skill to look after them, and equally the amount of support that he got from psychiatric colleagues, albeit how *willing* they were, was ludicrous because again the number of psychiatrists we have in relationship to any measure of population is quite small. So that the *main* objective which we hoped would happen, is that we would hopefully avoid the same number of patients presenting for admission to hospital, whether it be for a geriatric bed or for a psychiatric bed.

Some day hospital staff are of the opinion that the day hospital has resulted in the redirection of some psychogeriatric referrals which would previously have been inappropriately referred to the geriatric services. A medical officer, in his capacity as a GP, explained what he saw to be the effect of the day hospital on the psychogeriatric and geriatric sectors of care:

> INTERVIEWER: 'Do you find that the day hospital provides an alternative for a wide range of patients who come under the psychogeriatric category or is it more limited?'
>
> GP: 'No I have referred quite a few psychogeriatric patients to [the consultant] and he has been quite happy to take them. Its a different kettle of fish if you are looking for an in-patient bed. I don't think its really cut down the pressure on hospital beds – eh – I don't know, but I doubt that it has.'
>
> INTERVIEWER: 'I don't know of any direct evidence of the effect it is having.'
>
> GP: 'The only thing that might be – I don't think it's cut down the demand in psychogeriatric beds. Probably increased it, probably taken the pressure off Dr H and the geriatric beds. Patients who would previously have been referred to Dr H are now being referred to the day hospital.'
>
> INTERVIEWER: 'I find that very interesting. You're saying that the psychogeriatric day hospital has probably cut down the pressure on the geriatric beds?'
>
> GP: 'Yes.'
>
> INTERVIEWER: 'How does that happen?'
>
> GP: 'Dr H in the past took a lot of patients who weren't really geriatric. They were referred to him because there was absolutely nowhere in the psychogeriatric side that might be able to take them. I think however there has been a bit more turnover with the day hospital and [the consultant] in relation to the psychogeriatric beds, especially here.'

Nevertheless throughout our period of studying the hospital there remained a steady trickle of cases referred from the geriatric to the psychogeriatric sector on the grounds that there was a significant psychiatric component to the patient's problems. For example, a GP reported in referring one case:

> Increasingly antisocial behaviour. Behaving oddly. Spitting on the floor. Family have approached GP for hospital admission for both patient and his wife. Dr H

> [consultant geriatrician] visited on Monday. He arranged to take Mrs I for a fortnight from [the middle] of this month. He could do nothing for patient and requested psychogeriatric assessments.

Again, a letter from a consultant physician in geriatric medicine to the day hospital consultant reads:

> I visited this lady at home ... she is physically well but very demented. She is supported at home by her daughter who wishes to continue her care and by neighbours. I have referred her also to [a senior social worker] and he is arranging home help and possibly voluntary visiting also. We are admitting her to hospital [for two weeks] for a respite admission but I wondered if following this she might attend the day hospital. I gather there is a patient from [the same town] already attending and they might go together. I shall be grateful for your help.

Only occasionally are cases treated within both geriatric and psychogeriatric sectors at the same time. The following is a rare example. The consultant physician in geriatric medicine wrote:

> It would seem that in May 1979 she had a small stroke resulting in some left-side weakness ... since then her niece has been visiting regularly and both she and her husband are finding this too trying. She has had leg ulcers all her life which the district nurse attends to, failing eyesight and swollen legs. She is reported to be eating well and to be continent. I think she is deserving of admission for a couple of weeks to relieve the situation at home. She would in my opinion be very suitable for the day hospital and perhaps Dr McR would be willing to admit her for a short spell to one of his beds at Park Hospital to relieve the situation at home. I would however like to see her here at the clinic for assessment of her physical condition.

This trickle of referrals is matched by a similarly small number of referrals from the day hospital to the geriatric service. These are, for the most part, referrals which the day hospital considers to have been initially inappropriately referred to a psychogeriatric service.

In general terms, then, movement between the geriatric and psychogeriatric sectors is limited. It is likely that the day hospital has reduced the number of psychogeriatric cases inappropriately referred to the consultant geriatrician but the day hospital is also probably slightly increasing the demand on the geriatric services by attracting into the system referrals which might not otherwise have been made and then passing them on to the geriatric service. In any case the number of patients involved in all of these transfers is very small and our central conclusion is that the day hospital has made very little difference to the comparatively rigid boundaries which exist between the geriatric and psychogeriatric systems of care. If what is meant by the day hospital making an active contribution to the geriatric services is that the two services should be more closely co-ordinated in order to improve the overall efficiency of health services, then the day hospital has probably made no significant contribution on this count.

Domiciliary services

Other services with which the day hospital has contact are the domiciliary services provided by the social work department and the health board. Staff point to the importance of co-ordination and co-operation between the services and to the quality of the relationships which have been built up between these services and the day hospital. A nurse explained:

> Well I think now we are more in touch with home-help services – and with district nurses – than we ever were, y'know because of the – its like a link between the outside services and the hospitals, it used to be, it was very much 'them' and 'us' situation.

As well as improving communication between the hospital and domiciliary services, staff also point to the fact that the day hospital makes a direct contribution to reducing the workload of these services. A nurse made this point:

> I think we help the services outside as well, the district nursing services, the home-help services as well, because we can give them information, we can relieve some of the work of the district nurses. If we've the patient in here and there's dressing and bathing etc. to be done we can in some cases take that over. That gives them more time and relieves them as well.

Certainly we came across numerous examples, both in our sample and in discussion at the Tuesday meeting, of fruitful co-operation between the home-help service in particular and day hospital support for patients. For example, in one case the social background report reads:

> Due to Mr T's memory state it was impossible to get any information regarding his past history. All information therefore was accrued from the home-help organizer. As far as can be ascertained, Mr T has been living on his own for some years and was an independent and active man. However his memory of time and place is now so bad that he is incapable of managing his own affairs. His pension is collected by the home help. She buys all his requirements and banks any money left over. Apparently if Mr T is given any money he buys whisky in bulk, drinks it, is rendered incapable, losing control of his bodily functions etc. and on one occasion he cut through the TV cable. He also cut the cable from the electric razor, attempted to put the two bare ends of wire into the socket. Mr T is ambulant and continent and appears to be fairly physically fit for his age.
>
> Due to the isolation of this man, the obvious risk he is to himself and his neighbours, it would again be appropriate to give this man twenty-four-hour care. However if the bed situation will not allow this I would consider that he be recommended a place in the day hospital. This will enable us to keep a closer eye on this apparently deteriorating situation.

Whereas such cases might previously have been the subjects of demand by the home-help service for in-patient beds, the day hospital staff were (at least in some cases) in a position to help. Likewise the day hospital is heavily dependent in some cases upon the home help and other domiciliary services for the maintenance of the patients in their own homes. For example, the part which the home-help service plays in getting patients ready in the morning when the bus picks them up to bring them to the hospital is important in preparing patients for the journey and in the smooth running of transport arrangements. Likewise there are a number of occasions on which, faced with an immediate difficulty, the home helps have contacted the hospital and the social worker has immediately visited the home to deal with the troublesome situation.

Throughout our research we gained the distinct impression that the contribution which the day hospital makes to the home-help service, and the contribution which the home-help service makes to the running of the day hospital, constitutes a very good example of the way in which resources may be efficiently used and, we suspect, net levels of service provision increased. The quality of this relationship between services is in quite marked contrast to the quality of relationship either between the day hospital and the geriatric or the day-hospital and the social work services.

However not all domiciliary services relate as well to the hospital as does, apparently, the home-help service. For example, district nurses expected patients attending the day hospital to be bathed at the hospital whereas the hospital nurses do not expect to have to perform this task routinely. They consider that the district nurses should continue to look after patients in this way. This is an example of a point which we have made earlier. In admitting a patient the day hospital does not thereby see itself as totally responsible for patient care. Other services (in this case district nursing but in other cases social work or the GP) are expected to continue support. The relationship between the hospital and the home-help service seems to work relatively smoothly because both services have much to gain by the contribution which they can make to each other. Difficulties arise when a reciprocal relationship is not in the mutual interests of the parties involved.

Conclusion

Although the study is not a study of the overall system of care for the elderly mentally infirm, it has produced material which allows us to comment on relationships between the day hospital and related services. This chapter began by drawing upon our interview data to show the strength of the view that the services of the day hospital are justified, not only in terms of their impact upon patients and relatives directly, but also in terms of impact on other services. Throughout the rest of the chapter we set a variety of data against this view.

Our general conclusion has been that relationships between the day hospital and related services vary considerably. We discussed in turn the day hospital and general practice, field and residential social work, the rest of the psychiatric system, Park Hospital, the geriatric service and domiciliary services. In some instances our data are consistent with the claim that the day hospital is a success as measured by its impact upon the operation of other services. However, in some areas at least the day hospital appears simply to have taken over resources from other services and while these resources are being used effectively they have not made any net contribution to the overall performance of the services from the clients' relatives' point of view. From an evaluative perspective, our data also suggest that, on some crucial problems of interface between different sectors of the system of care for the elderly mentally infirm, the day hospital has achieved little. Indeed there are some crucial problems of relationship between organizations and professions which have been largely evaded by the way in which the hospital operates.

In drawing these conclusions about the success of the day hospital in its impact on, and relationships with, related services, we have, throughout the chapter, followed a line of discussion which has been consistent with our discussions of patient flow and other criteria of success. Outcomes very much depend upon the interests of the groups involved. The real difficulties arise because in many cases it is not in the interest of any major group within the day hospital to contribute significantly to an outside service. Overall the day hospital has done little to resolve the long-standing problems in service co-ordination which exist in the field of care for the elderly mentally infirm. In that sense the day hospital may be less of a radical initiative in its impact on related services than the culture of the hospital is inclined to imply.

CHAPTER NINE

Success as Relative Support: The Relatives' Views

Introduction

It is widely reported in the research literature that relatives of psychogeriatric patients play an important part in providing care and support for patients living at home (Isaacs, et al. 1972; Bergmann et al. 1978; see also Tinker 1981). The burden of care places considerable stress on families and there is increasing recognition of the need to provide services which 'support the supporters' (Hemsi 1982; Sheldon 1984; Allen et al. 1983b; Levin et al. 1983). Amongst day hospital staff there is a very widespread consensus on the importance of providing a service to the relatives of patients. There is also a general view that this is one area of service in which the day hospital has accomplished a great deal.

In this chapter we examine relatives' experiences and assessment of those aspects of the hospital's service which staff describe as providing 'support for relatives'. The chapter rests heavily upon our interviews with relatives but draws upon other material as well and, especially, sets relatives' views against data from the staff interviews. Our central conclusions are that staff and relatives' perceptions diverge and that relatives' evaluation of the service can only be understood in the context of their perceptions of what constitutes the 'problem' with the patient. The chapter therefore begins by outlining relatives' construction of the nature of the 'problem'.

The 'problem'

When answering questions of the type, 'What is wrong with the patient?', relatives seldom rely solely on precise medical diagnoses. This may well indicate a lack of medical knowledge on their part but it does not mean that they are at a loss for an explanation. Rather it reflects the fact that diagnostic terms of this kind are largely irrelevant to relatives. What is important to them is a commonsense reason for the changes in their patient and also the prognosis. Some relatives do acquire information from their GP and use some expressions derived from medical terms – such as 'hardening of the arteries' and 'senile' – which carry some explanatory power for them. However, these 'medical explanations' are incorporated, with varying degrees of accuracy, into the commonsense accounts of ageing and physical degeneration which most relatives initially use in trying to account for abnormal behaviour on the part of the patient. These accounts entail a number of not necessarily consistent social, personal, genetic and moral factors such as: sudden severe illness, chronic illness, accidents, bereavement, loss of work, loss of social activities, too much hard work, too much mental strain, too socially isolated, a 'highly strung nature', too introverted, a family trait, and a spoiled and lazy nature. As one relative expressed it: 'Its just the mind's breakin' up before the body. Well to me idea of thinken' that is what it is. It's auld age of the head before the heart and that.'

Some loss of mental acuity with increasing age is considered normal by most relatives. It is only when the deterioration exceeds their expectations that they look for additional explanations. The idea of physical change – such as hardening of the arteries within the brain – may provide relatives with some additional explanation but is not, apparently, adequate in providing them with reasons for one individual suffering while others do not. Relatives therefore often look to the individual patient's history, a point which is illustrated in the following extract:

> INTERVIEWER: 'What is your understanding of what actually caused it?'
> MRS H: 'Oh I should think it is just senile decay and I think, possibly I keep harping back to this but I keep thinking if she had had more company it wouldn't have happened so quickly.'
> INTERVIEWER: 'Can I ask you again, I am pushing you a bit, what do you mean when you say it is senile decay?'
> MRS H: 'Just the fact that her mental processes are slowing down because of old age, because of the deterioration that takes place in some people – it doesnae happen with everybody and you sometimes wonder why it doesn't, why it should happen even with my mother, in fact anybody's mother, why it should happen to some folk and doesn't happen to others. But a lot of it, I think, you see my mum had six of a family and she had a busy, busy life she really had ... she spent half her life at the stove and the other half washing, she had a busy, busy life and then suddenly there was nothing, well not suddenly, but over a shortish period she had nothing, so I can understand that.'

Not all relatives are the same. There are some differences between relatives of depressed patients and those suffering from dementia. The relatives of patients in our sample with a diagnosis of depression usually used the term 'depressed' in describing the patient but explained the depression as the consequence of physical illness resulting, in their account, either from physical discomfort associated with the illness or from the anxiety that the illness might be serious or even terminal. These relatives were not inclined to look to the individual's life history for explanation as did the relatives of dementia patients. (However, generally the numbers are very small and the position might well have been different had a larger number of depression cases, including some without physical problems, occurred in the sample.)

Further differences between dementia cases and depressed cases are reflected in relative's views about prognosis. Relatives of patients diagnosed as suffering from dementia hold a very pessimistic view and foresee no serious possibility of improvement. This is true whether or not the relatives have any medical knowledge of the diagnosis.

So far as the problem itself is concerned (as distinct from explanation or prognosis) relatives experience and describe a very wide range of patient incapacities and behaviours which they regard as departing from the 'normal' for their patient. These include general forgetfulness, aggression, wandering, incontinence, inability to cope with various activities of daily living, sleep disturbance, risk with electricity, gas, or fires, mood disturbance, hallucinations, and inability to communicate. A full list of aspects of the problem mentioned by relatives is set out in Figure 7. This list compares closely with other studies of the problems reported by carers of psychogeriatric patients (Wheatley 1980; Gilliard and Watt

Sight problems
Hearing impairment
Restricted mobility
Weight problem
Inactivity
Restlessness and agitation
Loss of interest and concentration
Inability to hold conversation
Telling 'stories' and lies
Not wanting company
Swearing
Bad table manners
Wandering
Forgetfulness
Delusions
Aggressiveness
Violence
Bad temper
Depression
'Funny moods'
Irrational fears
'Carnapcious'
Incontinence
Bad toilet behaviour
Unreasonably demanding
Hallucinations
Poor hygiene
Dirty habits
Not recognizing people
Disorientation in time
Losing things, especially money
Irresponsibility with money
Taking other people's belongings
Obsessions
Sleep disturbance
Refusing to go to bed
Hiding things, especially money
Getting lost, including within the home
Eating and drinking inappropriate things
Dressing inappropriately
Refusing to dress
Dangerous behaviour with fires, cookers and cigarettes
No longer managing cooking, housework, shopping and cleaning
Refusing medication
Complaining of physical symptoms

Figure 7 Aspects of the 'problem' mentioned by relatives.

1982). However our experience in interviewing alerted us to the possibility of interpreting these data in a way which is at variance with some previous research.

There is a tendency in studies of the problems of family support to imply that the difficulties which patients present can be related to the seriousness of the problems which carers experience (Greene et al. 1982). We found that relatives themselves often had difficulty in ordering patient characteristics according to any notion of the severity of the problems for the family. Initially we did ask relatives to rank those aspects of the patient's condition which presented problems for them. But typically relatives would select only one or two 'worst' characteristics. They would describe these in considerable detail, often with long accounts of specific incidents. If more than one relative was present there was likely to be some disagreement between them. If pressed to comply with the task that we had set, some respondents were prepared to oblige but we quickly concluded that what was being asked of them did not reflect the way in which they conceived of the problem. Caring for the relative was not a matter of individual gradeable difficulties arising from specific symptoms. We suspect that the precise scaling techniques used in some other studies are not a valid reflection of the relatives' own way of thinking.

So, to judge from our data, the extent to which patients constitute a problem for relatives is only partially dependent on specific incapacities or behaviours (Daatland 1982) and there is no direct relationship between the problem for the relative and the number of incapacities presented. For relatives construe the 'problem' in terms of the *overall social situation* in which they find themselves. Thus specific patient difficulties mean different things to different relatives depending upon the implications for them in their particular setting.

The following extract from one interview is illustrative of the kind of data on which we based these conclusions. The response followed questioning about the deterioration in the patient's condition. The respondent is the patient's daughter, who lives next door to her father and who shares care with her sister who lives nearby.

> Oh aye he was really – in the hoose himsel putting the gases all on and wasnae putting a light to them. See I used to go up first thing in the morning before the home help came. I had his breakfast by before she came in cause she couldnae come to 9 o'clock. And I used ta say 'Oh my, there is a smell of gas' and to me he even tried to make himself something but it has been in his mind 'I'm hungry and ah want a cup of tea' and he has went and he's all terribly confused with everything he done. . . . He put sugar on the top o' a piece of ham that wasnae cooked and a slice of bread and it was a' just sitting in the oddest places. I went up one morning and this is what he done – of course this is really queer. When I went up I said to myself you must have been feeling hungry and he has made the effort to put the bacon in the pan but he hasnae even went to the cooker wi'it. It has been in his mind 'I'll make something' and – here I thought it was fat at first, the fat in the bottom of the pan y'know was, you could see it hadnae been melted or nothing and it was really white looking and this stuff that was roon it looked like fat but seemed to be squirmed roun it and I said how could that be different from that if that is cold y'know. An I looked aboot the workshop and, he has got this cream

> that he got for his psorasis in big tubes that [the GP] gied him. There was a tube cut in half and he must have squirted that all roond it and that is whit it wa. I says of my Goad he'll get poisoned – but I mean he hadnae cooked it but he could ha'. As I say he didnae know where the toilet was and he kept his ash pail in the kitchen and he was going in and he was using that as the toilet. More or less it was on the flair than it was in the pail and some mornings he was dirty which I couldnae clean up and in the feenish up J. [sister] had to dae that. I had to wait till she came up and I says J. you have got a mess to clear up because I couldnae dae it. And when you went up on the morning he was up and the covers were up on his bed and it was all kind of bumptied and I pulled the cover back and there ma father had his shoes, his jackets, shirts all in this, in his bed. Even I went up one day and he had the electric fan heater on the tap o' his bed y'ken inside it. It wasnae on or anything like that I just couldnae make head or tail of what he was trying tae dae. And you would say to him 'Right Dad, come on and get ready'. Father would mebbe be sitting with one sock on as you thought. There was one sock but he had the two socks on the one fit and nae sock on the other one. Things like that he was just getting worse every day. When you went up he had done something else but it was never him, he didnae know he was daeing it.

The 'social situation' of the relatives, as we have described it, variously comprises the relatives' own health and personal routines, immediate family relationships, the relationship between relative and patient, social activities, employment, relationships with friends and neighbours, the extended family network and the relatives' image of themselves as competent caring family members. So, for example, the difficulties which carers experience vary considerably depending upon whether or not they are themselves elderly and frail or suffering from some form of chronic illness. In the area of domestic routines the biggest problem for relatives is not an increase in workload as such but rather disruption to existing patterns caused by caring for the patient. The extent to which the carer perceives the patient as a problem varies too with the impact of care upon other members of the carer's immediate family. This impact varies, in turn, with the quality of pre-existing family relationships. The extent to which relatives perceive the patient as having an adverse effect on their social activities depends on the limits which the demands of patient care place upon what the carer regards as a 'normal' social life. Also the employment position of the carer is very important. For example, the perception of one respondent who was unemployed but looking for work was very different from the perception of another respondent who recently had willingly given up part-time work in order to remain at home and care for her mother.

We conclude, on the basis of our interview material, therefore, that although the patient's 'clinical' condition is significant it is the overall 'social situation' which constitutes the 'problem' for relatives. This perspective is different from that which is characteristic of day hospital staff (and we should also bear in mind at this point 'the hospital's definition of the problem', as we described it in Chapter 6). So service intervention will only be successful, from the relatives' point of view, if it directly improves their social situation as they define it. In the next section we suggest that relatives' views, on the success of the day hospital's services in providing them with support, can be understood in the light of this argument.

The service

We explained that a service to relatives is one major criterion which is used to assess the success of the day hospital. Staff suggest that the following features are specifically important:

(1) Frequent contact is maintained between hospital and home.
(2) Relatives are relieved of the burden of care by removal of the patient from the home for set periods (custodial care).
(3) The hospital provides relatives with a source of advice on patient management and care.
(4) Relatives themselves receive emotional support and therapy from the hospital.

We now compare staff views on these points with the reactions of relatives (For comparative studies of relatives' reactions to various forms of day provision, see Brocklehurst and Tucker 1980; Fennell et al. 1981; and Gilliard and Watt 1982). We consider first the importance of contact between hospital and home.

Contact between hospital and home
Many members of staff stress that knowledge of the home background and patients' progress there is important. It is a prerequisite to action both in planning individual treatment programmes, and in allowing the day hospital to respond to family needs. Staff generally think that good communication does exist with relatives. They point to the fact that relatives are welcome to visit the hospital, that nursing escorts who accompany the patients on the bus have frequent contact with family members and that the relatives' group additionally provides an important opportunity for staff and family members to meet.

The most obvious channel of communication between the day hospital and family is the patient who moves between the two settings regularly. In practice however, as relatives and staff pointed out, the patient may be an extremely unreliable source of information, especially if they are confused and their memory impaired. Many are even unware that they have attended the hospital and it can be difficult to obtain very simple pieces of information from the patient. The daughters of two patients explained this problem. First:

> INTERVIEWER: 'What's been your mother's reaction to attending the day hospital?'
> MRS H: 'I don't think there is one, if she even realizes she's been there.'
> INTERVIEWER: 'Nothing at all?'
> MRS H: 'No nothing, absolutely nothing.'
> INTERVIEWER: 'It is never mentioned.'
> MRS H: 'You may say, "Had you a good day today?" and she just looks at you blankly.'

And in the second case:

> MISS T: 'Well, if we say to her when she comes in, "What did you have for your lunch?" she can't remember. "What did you do today?" "Oh! I don't know!".'

Staff suggest that a solution to this difficulty lies with the escorts who provide a valuable means of communication. Relatives describe these contacts as fleeting because the escorts must hurry to collect all the patients within a limited time. One patient's husband resented this haste:

> MR X: 'Everybody's in a hurry. Everybody wants to go, there's nobody got time. Even when they came to take her away I used to say to the nurse, "For God's sake nurse don't push her around like that." She says, "I've got a time schedule, I have got other patients to lift." I mean you don't have to carry on like that (c'mon, c'mon, c'mon) – they have all got to go by the watch.'

However, in spite of the fact that many relatives referred to the brevity of the contacts, such complaints about the tone of the interaction are few. Relatives more often commented with gratitude on the skill and patience of the escorts in persuading reluctant patients to attend. However, several relatives pointed out that nursing escorts do not generally initiate discussions about the patient's condition and progress which are the subjects of greatest concern to relatives. Few relatives actually expected much detailed personal discussion both because of the circumstances of the interaction and because of the low status of the staff involved. Generally, then, when this does occur, conversation between relatives and the escorts tends to consist simply of social chitchat and generalized enquiries. The daughter of one patient explained:

> INTERVIEWER: 'With your father going back and forward in the bus do you have any contact with the nurses?'
> MRS N: 'Well you usually get the one in the morning to come in and sort of pass the time of day and ask if they have been on holiday and things like that – but not really an awful lot of contact with them.'
> INTERVIEWER: 'So you don't really have a chance to talk to them much about how he is getting on?'
> MRS N: 'No. Sometimes when they bring him home I say, "How was he today?" – "Oh well a wee bit confused and unsettled". But that's all they ever say. Of course it'll no be their place to stay anything I don't suppose.'

The staff viewpoint also overlooks the fact that many relatives do not live with the patient and therefore have no regular contact with escorts. In these cases this means of communication breaks down completely.

In the eyes of most relatives, detailed personal consultation about the patient would, anyway, more appropriately take place with medically qualified staff and many would welcome the opportunity to discuss their patient's case with the consultant at the day hospital. The following exchange summarizes many relatives' feelings:

> INTERVIEWER: 'Do you have much contact with nurses that collect her on the bus or bring her back?'
> MRS N: 'O aye.'
> INTERVIEWER: 'Does that give much opportunity to tell you what is happening?'
> MRS N: 'No. I don't know whether it is because they are auxiliaries. I just havenae, I have never actually ... I'll ask [the nurse] "How did she get on today?" and she'll say, "Oh she got kind of nervous today and she wouldnae sit doon. She

got on fine!" They have always made a wee comment, but I have actually sort of asked them any . . .'

INTERVIEWER: 'Would you think it is not appropriate to ask them about medication and prescriptions and things like that?'

MRS N: 'That's right and I don't know whether they are on shifts too. The one that collects her in the mornings is no the one that brings her back so they are only on sort of half day. I would like to talk, in fact I would like to talk to the doctor to – and see what's happening and how long this is going on for . . .'

In practice the only point in the patient's career at which the relatives routinely have contact with senior day hospital staff is when the patient is being considered for admission. Although many relatives do have a discussion with the consultant or the social worker (or occasionally both), at this stage the arrangements for meeting relatives tend to be rather haphazard. It is not unusual for relatives who play a key role in patient care not to have had this opportunity, especially if they live some distance away from the patient. Thereafter opportunities are seldom *provided* for relatives to meet the consultant.

The social worker on the other hand is generally more accessible to relatives but again contact is not maintained with relatives on a routine basis. It is initiated at times of crisis or when some specific arrangements are being made (for example a holiday admission to in-patient care). There was only one family interviewed who received the kind of direct social work assistance that might be considered to constitute extended casework. In this case the social worker was involved in assisting one relative in making arrangements for care of the patient to be shared with her rather reluctant sisters. The arrangements lasted only a short time but the relative was nevertheless grateful for the social worker's intervention which she saw as significant in bringing about greater family involvement. Other relatives specifically mentioned that they would have liked more contact with the social worker, especially in discussing the patient's discharge and the availability of follow-up services.

In other respects, too, staff views about contact between hospital and home are at variance with the relatives' experience. Although staff emphasize that relatives are welcome to visit the day hospital at any time, in practice this does not happen very frequently. Two of the relatives interviewed regularly took their patients along to the hospital by car but these were exceptions. Many of the relatives interviewed had never visited the hospital. Apart from those who had gone to the relatives' group, the relatives we spoke to who had visited the day hospital had done so for a very specific and exceptional reason; for example, taking the patient in late on an occasion when they had overslept and the patient had missed the bus. Most relatives found it difficult to visit the day hospital because of transport difficulties and other commitments, yet many felt that they were themselves to blame for the lack of contact with staff. Relatives who did visit the hospital generally had very limited conversations with staff and did not find full and detailed personal consultation.

The only routine occasion on which relatives visit the day hospital is to attend the relatives' group, but there are considerable difficulties which prevent many relatives from attending the group and for this and other reasons it does not generally solve the problem of communication between hospital and home. The group is an extremely important feature of the hospital's attempt to provide a 'service to relatives' and is therefore dealt with in detail in the next chapter. However, an important point to note here is that the group has unintended consequences for relatives who do not attend. These relatives note that hospital staff arrange the group as an occasion for them to go along and meet staff. If they do not accept this invitation they feel that they have forfeited their opportunity and they do not feel justified thereafter in complaining about lack of information about the hospital or their patient. The following is a comment from one relative, a Mrs T: '. . . Well we don't know. Of course its my fault not goin' over, when you've got a night to be over. I've never been over.' The son of another patient expressed similar views:

> INTERVIEWER: 'Have there been any problems with her actually going to the day hospital, getting her there and things . . .'
> MR M: 'Not to my knowledge. I haven't had any contact – obviously that's my fault as well, because they have meetings.'
> INTERVIEWER: 'Do you know very much about what happens at the day hospital with her?'
> MR M: 'I know nothing really about that.'

In a small number of cases relatives had little interest in finding out about the day hospital or the patient's progress. Several factors contribute to this. Firstly some relatives with a pessimistic view of the patient's condition can see no point in meeting staff merely to have this view confirmed. Secondly some relatives take the view that it is best to 'let the experts get on with their job'. In the face of professional skills they feel that they can make no contribution to planning or administering treatment. For example:

> INTERVIEWER: 'Do you feel you would like to have known a bit more?'
> MRS N: 'Well I don't know – I feel they are trained for the job and I leave it in their hands. That's the way I look at it, they will know more about it than I will know about it.'

Finally a minority of relatives who are peripherally or reluctantly involved in patient care are resistant to any activities which make further demands on their time.

Custodial care

As we have said, staff also suggest that the day hospital provides a service to relatives by offering relief through custodial care. Certainly many relatives feel that they benefit directly from having the patient away at the day hospital for set periods and custodial care is important to relatives in a number of ways.

Firstly having their patient in a safe and secure environment for specified periods relieves the relatives of anxiety about mishaps which could otherwise arise. The daughter of one patient explained:

> INTERVIEWER: 'From your point of view, what do you think of the day hospital?'
> MRS H: Well I can see that they are doing a lot of good work for a lot of people and it is a help to me, I couldn't say anything else. For two working days I know

my mother is being looked after all the time I am at work. There is no danger of a fire or anything like that. So I think that's marvellous.'

This kind of relief is particularly, though not exclusively, associated with cases where the relative does not actually live with the patient. But relatives living with patients are also able to use the time to get on with domestic chores and other tasks which are difficult when the patient's needs have constantly to be kept in mind. Moreover the opportunity to get on with domestic chores in the patient's absence may produce benefits in allowing the relative to concentrate on providing a better standard of care for the patient at other times. A relative explained:

INTERVIEWER: 'Is it important that she still goes to the day hospital do you think?'
MR McH: 'Oh aye, because it gives me a rest. I mean that's her awa' for the day and I can go doon the toon. I can dae whatever I have to dae. Wednesday I walk up to [the supermarket] and get my messages [shopping], then I can get things done up the stair that I cannae get done when she is here because I want to gie her a wee bit company that you cannae just have her sitting here like a dummy.'

And at another point in the interview:

MR McH: ... This is the way the day hospital is great for me because through the day I havenae got her through the day that I can cope better at night. But see when you have got it all day and all night and nobody else in the hoose that's the problem ...

And finally, the break quite simply gives relatives a chance to unwind:

MRS H: '... so it was a great help. You've nae idea the relief it is to know she'll be all right, and you're gettin' a couple of hours where you can sit down and relax ...'

Overall, relatives point to relief by custodial care as the main benefit to be derived from the hospital.

However, custodial care has its limitations. Firstly, difficulties in coping with patients during the night are fairly common. Obviously the day hospital can do nothing to help patients' families here. As one relative, Mrs H, made the point: 'But I think that's a good idea this day care centre – just to take a bit o' the worry off ye, albeing you've the worry coming back at night. Because it is a worry. It really is.' Secondly, there is the serious limitation, from the relatives' point of view, that attendance must be discontinued if the patient is physically unwell for a short time or physically deteriorates to such an extent that transport on the coach is no longer possible. For many relatives such physical complications add considerably to their burden. The day hospital service is thus being withdrawn at a time when the relatives' need for it has increased. Thirdly, a limitation for relatives is that the service is usually only provided for two or three days per week. Relatives who feel that they benefit from the patient's attendance would often welcome an increase in the number of days. However most relatives are aware that resources are limited and often evaluate the service in this light. There is certainly a strong sense of 'anything is better than nothing', as this extract shows:

> INTERVIEWER: 'Your mother hasn't been attending the day hospital very long but what's your opinion so far of the service that's being offered there?'
> MRS H: 'I think it's good, it definitely is good, aye. Because as I say, I know where she is and I know she's under supervision. I know she's no gettin' doin' somethin' that may be could harm hersel' – oh – its a relief for me as well as for her.'
> INTERVIEWER: 'Do you think it's enough?'
> MRS H: 'Well – it's maybe no enough but it's a good help. It might no' be enough but it's certainly a good help. It's better than nothin' lets put it that – it's an *awful* lot better than nothin' – it's 100 better than nothing. As I say, whether it's enough or not I don't know. I don't know whether sometimes they make it more than two days a week. I don't know. If they did I would be perfectly happy for my mother to go more than two days a week . . .'

Fourthly, day hospital attendance incurs costs as well as benefits for some relatives and these costs must be taken into account in assessing the effectiveness of the service. While some relatives see a direct relationship between the number of days attendance and the benefit accrued this is not applicable in cases where attendance creates extra work for the relative. Difficulties, often connected with getting the patient ready to go, arise particularly in cases where the relative is also elderly and perhaps frail. In some cases day hospital attendance may so aggravate the situation at home that the relatives, on balance, experience little benefit. The husband of one patient explained:

> INTERVIEWER: 'Was the day hospital much help to you at that stage [when the patient was frail]?'
> MR X: 'No! Not a bit! They in their wisdom thought it would be much better for *me* to get a day but it took an awful lot out of me to get her ready for it.'
> INTERVIEWER: 'They thought it would be better for you that Mrs X was going away for the day.'
> MR X: 'They thought that taking her away – "Oh look at the lovely day you will have, you can do what you like, you know," and that sort of thing. I was exhausted getting her ready because I had to start about 6 o'clock in the morning to get her tuned in sort of thing and to talk her into it because she didn't want to go and sometimes she would just sit there half-dressed. It's an awful job to dress a woman.' [Laughs]
> INTERVIEWER: 'You didn't feel you got much of a break with having her there?'
> MR X: 'No, not at all. By the time she would leave here [it was] about twenty-to-nine and I got her away I had everything to tidy up and go out and get something for the dinner. I was exhausted – and before I knew where I was it was half-past two or something and she was due home about half past three.'

Thus if the day hospital is to provide maximum benefit to relatives, account must be taken of any additional demands which attendance may create and services must be provided to compensate for them. So far as custodial care is concerned we must be careful not to presume that, from the relatives' standpoint, 'more' in terms of time *necessarily* means 'better' in terms of relief.

Advice on patient care

The emphasis which staff place on the day hospital as a means of educating relatives in better methods of patient care was not reflected in the comments which relatives made about their experiences of the service. Very few of them mentioned advice from the hospital on patient care as significant. The relatives' group does provides some relatives with limited assistance (as we shall describe) but other relatives felt that they had not learned from the day hospital about how they might better cope with their patient. Any advice that was received was inclined to be viewed as 'common sense' rather than the application of professional or technical expertise. As one relative expressed this in interview:

> INTERVIEWER: 'What about getting advice about how to cope with the problems? Has the day hospital been any help with that?'
>
> MRS N: 'No really. I can't find that they have, no I really couldnae say that, I mean I feel as if well anything they have said I have known that on my own or managed to cope with it on my own, but as far as that goes, no it certainly didnae make any difference whatever.'

Emotional support

Staff also suggest that day hospital intervention provides relatives with emotional support and has the effect of improving their coping capacities and their adjustment to their situation. The only references by relatives to the day hospital's help in meeting their psychological and emotional needs (other than by providing custodial care) were in connection with the relatives' group, which was viewed as a source of some emotional support.

> INTERVIEWER: 'Did the day hospital do much to help you?'
>
> MRS H: 'Well I felt that the relatives' support group did help because at least you could get speaking about it and you were mixing with somebody that had the same problems . . .'

Yet even with the group, relatives report limitations, as we shall see.

Conclusion

In this chapter we have dealt with two interlinked themes. First, we have described how relatives define their problem with the patient in the context of their particular social situation. Second, we have described the rather diverging views between staff and relatives about the hospital's success in providing relative support. The operation of the day hospital is based upon assumptions about the nature of the problem for relatives which are generally not shared by the relatives themselves. The hospital focuses its main efforts on the patients rather than on resolving family difficulties, and hospital services do not respond to individual family circumstances and needs in ways which relatives regard as effective. Consequently the day hospital has comparatively little impact on the 'problem' *as this is construed by relatives* – that is, on their difficult social situation.

At several points through the chapter we have mentioned the relatives' group as an important aspect of the day hospital's support for relatives. We devote the next chapter specifically to this topic.

CHAPTER TEN

Success as Relative Support: The Relatives' Group

Introduction

A relatives' group in which the social worker attached to the hospital plays a leading role, is a major component of the service which the day hospital offers to relatives of patients. Even though systematic liaison with relatives did not form any major part in the planning and design of the organization as a whole, and even though the group remains comparatively self-contained and is organized somewhat separately from the main body of hospital activities, its meetings represent the few occasions on which relatives have regular contact with hospital staff. This chapter therefore continues our assessment of the success of the day hospital on the criterion of relative support by presenting data specifically concerned with the activities of this group. We shall describe its major features, comment on the part that it plays within the day hospital as a whole and discuss the way in which it serves different constituent interests in different ways.

To anticipate our conclusions, we shall suggest that the relatives' support group sustains an ideology of service to relatives while nevertheless confining many of the practical tasks so entailed to a self-contained and rather isolated organizational locale. This minimizes the problems of 'relative disturbance' to the rest of the institution.

Apart from its relevance to an evaluation of the day hospital, there are implications of this thesis for professional practice, particularly for social work in medicine. Insofar as social workers play a significant part in running such groups, their attempts to introduce relatives in this way as significant consumers may, ironically, serve only to limit their impact within the system of medical care.

Major features of the group

The provision of assistance to relatives of patients by means of a support group was not envisaged as an integral part of the service when the day hospital was being planned. The idea was not formulated until after the day hospital became operational the initiative originating from the newly appointed staff. The social worker and sister-in-charge were key figures in promoting this development although other members of staff, including the senior enrolled nurse, the community nurse and secretary, were also involved from a very early stage. The staff of the day hospital itself was generally very enthusiastic about the concept of providing a support group for relatives but administrative staff, who had responsibility for the day hospital amongst other services, showed some caution. This type of involvement with relatives entailed, for them, a departure from the customary model of hospital services in which relatives play no significant part and boundaries between the institution and the home are clearly defined and maintained. Their reservations about this innovation in service to relatives took the form of raising issues such as whether the group should be permitted to meet on hospital premises, whether nursing staff should receive payment for attending evening sessions, the right of senior nursing staff to 'drop in' on the proceedings at will, and the position with regard to any funds raised by the group. Despite the expression of such concerns by the administrative staff, which caused considerable friction in the formative stages of the group, there was no effective opposition on their part and they eventually accommodated the group as a feature of the day hospital service.

The first meetings of the group took place about four months after the day hospital opened. To begin with, a group meeting was held on one afternoon and one evening of every second week. It was hoped that, by having an evening meeting, relatives who worked would be able to participate. After a few months the afternoon session was discontinued because it was very expensive on staff time. It was also difficult to arrange for visiting speakers to attend both sessions, and staff eventually came to the view that one bigger group would be more effective than two smaller groups. The group then continued, with holiday breaks, on the basis of a fortnightly evening meeting in the activity area of the day hospital. This provides a very comfortable setting, conducive to the informal atmosphere which the staff aim to create.

There is a strong shared sense that staff who attend should do so regularly. (At one time the attendance of a senior member of staff who wished to drop in on the group occasionally was resisted on the grounds that staff should be seen 'to be committed'). For the most part, staff who have attended have done so very regularly indeed. Typically those present are the sister-in-charge, the social worker, the senior enrolled nurse, the secretary and occupational therapist.

The pattern of the relatives' attendance is more irregular. At any one time, about 20% of patients have no relatives who could attend. Seldom are there relatives of more than 20% of patients attending. Our estimate is that, over time, for all patients admitted, a maximum of 30% have relatives who ever attend. Frequency, regularity and span of attendance vary considerably. Some relatives have attended on one occasion only. Others have maintained attendance regularly or spasmodically over a period of two years. In most cases relatives cease attending the group when the patient is discharged from the hospital but a few continue to attend after their patient is admitted to a long-term bed in Park Hospital.

Family members who attend the group are related to patients in various ways and come from varied family structures. We have no evidence that they are unrepresentative of the overall hospital population in these respects. Group members, who may or may not be co-resident with the patient, have included spouses, adult offspring (including those related by marriage), nieces and granddaughters. Women numerically predominate at the group as they do amongst supporters generally. Sometimes only one family member attends, but in other cases several relatives have come together. Most relatives who attend the group are very actively involved in the care of the patient and in this respect may be rather unrepresentative of the population of patients' relatives as a whole. However that is not to imply that non-attendance is an indicator of lesser involvement in patient care, as many relatives who are not group members are equally committed to the support of their patient and there are certainly a number of difficulties involved for many relatives in attending the group. We have mentioned that the day hospital is not readily accessible by public transport, and relatives come from a dispersed geographical area. (The hospital bus used for patients is not available for the relatives group.) Perhaps most important, relatives often have to arrange for a sitter for their patient. Indeed, for many the essence of their problem is that they cannot leave the patient alone. Rarely, patients have accompanied relatives to the group but this practice is not encouraged.

Typically, then, the group comprises five staff and about ten relatives, although on one occasion there was a group meeting at which twenty-four relatives were present while at the other extreme there have been evenings when staff have outnumbered relatives.

We shall be providing detailed material on the content of relatives' group meetings in a later section of this chapter but some general features of the events of a typical meeting can be summarized here. The relatives usually begin to arrive around 7 p.m. and are served with coffee while they chat with other relatives and staff. When it is clear that the majority of those expected have arrived and are seated in the circle of chairs arranged for the meeting, one of the staff members, usually the social worker, will suggest that they 'get started'. After a short period of introductions, general conversation about forthcoming events and so on, the focus of the discussion moves to individual cases. It is accepted by staff and relatives that this 'wee chat' involves going round the group and giving each relative in turn the opportunity to talk about their patient in detail. In this part of the meeting relatives are usually very open in recounting their experiences and frequently become emotional. However, there is also often a good deal of humour in their accounts of some of the incidents which have occurred with their patient. Although one might expect this kind of discussion to differ as between relatives who are spouses and relatives who are children, in practice this is not obviously so. Similarly one might expect men to be more reluctant to display their emotions in this semi-public setting. While a few men contribute comparatively little, many males are as vocal as their female counterparts.

The discussion tends to move back and forth between staff members and the relatives of any one patient but other relatives do join in with comments. More specifically, four features characterize these interactions. First, most exchanges consist essentially of a two-party interaction between a member of staff and a relative. Second, although when one relative 'holds the floor' other relatives do join in and are often actively brought in by staff to support their perspective, there remains nevertheless a distinct sense of 'turn taking' in the flow of discussion. Third, interaction is quite highly controlled. The levels of distress and aggression tolerated by staff and other relatives are limited. On the occasions when relatives appear to be exceeding these limits the rising tension is diffused by staff. Fourth, whatever the specifics of the exchange, there is a continual sense of staff presenting an account of the 'social reality' of the hospital regime, the ageing process, the role of relatives, or whatever, in a setting in which relatives either lack a framework of ideas with which to make sense of their position, or (as we have shown in Chapter 9) hold a perspective which is at variance to that which the hospital can accommodate.

Occasionally arrangements are made for a guest speaker to attend the group and in the past these have included representatives from the community health council, the electricity board, gas board, police and home-help service, as well as other medical and paramedical personnel such as the dietitian, a district nurse, sister-in-charge of one of the wards in Park Hospital and a nursing officer. Meetings vary on these occasions with some being entirely devoted to discussion of the material presented by the speaker. In others the latter part of the evening reverts to the usual format of discussion of individual cases. On two occasions the consultant psychiatrist in charge of the day hospital has attended.

For a small number of meetings films have been shown, either hired by staff or provided by relatives. Some have been holiday films unrelated to the work of the hospital but generally they have been connected in some way with the problems of the elderly and their relatives, and have served as starting points for discussion.

At intervals, meetings are devoted entirely to social gatherings such as a cheese and wine party. The group also has spent time planning and organizing fund-raising events in aid of additional facilities and activities for patients. The most prominent of these activities was a short weekend holiday for patients which was run mainly by staff but with relatives also participating.

The meetings usually last between two and two-and-a-half hours. The end of the meeting, as the beginning, is often indistinct with some relatives beginning to drift off early to fit in with transport and other arrangements. Eventually a member of staff may draw the meeting to a close with reminders about future plans, although often the group discussion simply disintegrates into a number of individual conversations while the relatives gradually take their leave.

Functions of the group

In the section that follows we outline the main categories of interaction which we have observed and the functions that the group meetings perform.

Exchange of information

First there is the exchange of practical information. The need for this arises because the patients themselves, although they are rarely considered to be reliable transmitters of practical intelligence, are the only regular channel of communication between staff and relatives. (We discussed the problem associated with nursing auxiliaries in this respect earlier.) Thus staff answer questions on the timing of bus journeys, the meals taken by patients, medication regimes and so on. Relatives frequently complain that the patients give them no account of what they have been doing at the hospital. The following extract from an annotated transcript of a group meeting illustrates this problem:

> SOCIAL WORKER [describing the group to new relatives]: '... But basically that is what we're [i.e. the group] about and usually what we do is we just sort of ask everybody what's been happening, what they're worried about, if there's anything puzzling you about the running of the thing, "Do they get fed?" and stuff like that ...'
>
> [Several relatives comment on changes in patients' eating habits since starting at the unit. Sister explains about meal times and how this ties in with the various transport times. Mrs N comments that she could not understand why her mother refused to eat when she came home from the day hospital. Now it is clear.]
>
> SISTER [to social worker]: 'It's just, remember that some relatives were wondering why the patients were bursting out of their dresses? [Laughter] It was because they were eating again, and again about nine o'clock.'
>
> SOCIAL WORKER: 'We didn't realize that everybody was – we thought everybody knew.'
>
> [Lots of comments from relatives merge – laughter.]
>
> 'And do you feel that she's benefiting from it all?' [to Mrs N.]
>
> MRS N: 'I don't know, she doesn't remember coming. You say: "How did you get on today?" – [she says] "How, where was I?" Just off the bus five minutes!'

Staff present information in a way that allows them to stress what they consider to be important about the day hospital, especially the rehabilitative nature of its services. For example, at one group meeting the following exchange took place:

> SISTER [responding to a relative's enquiry]: 'Each patient that comes to the department comes on an assessment basis; occupational therapy assessment, social work assessment, nursing assessment, medical assessment from Dr McD, the medical officer, and psychiatric assessment from Dr McR, the consultant. That period's usually a month, a month's assessment period where everybody's involved to get a full assessment of the patient and their capabilities, the first month they come.'
>
> SOCIAL WORKER: 'When they're being assessed, each week we have a weekly meeting with Dr McR and all the staff involved with the patient, and each patient

is discussed, how they are getting on, what's happening, something particular of concern ...'

MRS H: [She had been looking extremely tense throughout the meeting, not responding much to humour etc.] 'How do you find out what they are capable of doing at home? Whether or not they can make themselves a cup of tea, whether or not they can wash themselves when they get up in the morning, how do you ...?'

SOCIAL WORKER: [in response to this threat – this is not really her area]: 'Well we would find out. [The occupational therapist] would find out here in the bedroom, that she's not capable of dressing herself, or she's not capable of remembering that the cooker's on, or whatever. If there is such an alarm we would try to do something about that, or you may tell us before they ever get here, you may say to me, "She can't do that, she can't be left," as all of you do, you all tell me that kind of thing, so I come armed with that information at the start, but [the occupational therapist] and sister do their own assessment as they're going along, which reinforces whether or not what you've been saying is wrong or it's a lie, but yes she's as bad here as she is there. Sometimes they're better here ...'

[The occupational therapist had tried unsuccessfully to put her point of view during the social worker's speech.]

SISTER: 'We work on what you call the Crichton scaling rate, so we can actually measure the patient's improvement ... although you may think your own relative is so demented they can't be rehabilitated at all, but [the occupational therapist] and the nursing team can maybe work on her, so they can dress themselves if they've just got out of the habit of dressing themselves, if their memory recall is not very good reinforcing it all the time, that is a form of rehabilitation with them.'

For their part relatives provide information to staff on, for example, whether they are managing to bath patients, whether they are ensuring that the patient receives the correct medication, and how the patient is responding to this, whether the patient is eating properly at home, and the kind of transport arrangements required. Relatives also provide staff with information in response to questions about the condition and progress of patients, this often serving as the starting-point for negotiating an account of the nature of the patient's condition.

Both staff and relatives derive practical benefit from this exchange of information. However, while for staff it additionally provides an opportunity to present to relatives an image of the day hospital as an active therapeutically oriented institution, for relatives, the exchange of practical information is more often used as a starting-point for discussing their individual case. The interests of the two groups in this exchange of information differ somewhat.

Individual consultation

Staff attempt to generate an air of informality within the hospital which will encourage regular discussions about patients between relatives and staff. They point out to relatives, when the subject arises, that it is open to them to make a specific appointment to see either the consultant or the sister-in-charge. However, in practice this does not often occur. In Chapter 9 we pointed out that many relatives are not in regular contact with the hospital. The occasions on which they are contacted by staff (either during the preparations of initial reports or when nursing auxiliaries collect or return patients on the bus) do not, from the relatives' point of view, serve the functions of offering specific diagnosis, prognosis and advice on handling the patient. Thus relatives seek to use the occasion of the relatives' group for this purpose. The following field note reports one attempt to obtain individual advice:

> Mrs H said that her mother was getting a good diet and she wondered if she was getting too much. Sister said that she could put her on a 1,000-calorie diet, but the conversation was not specifically conclusive. In some ways these meetings are a very unsatisfactory form of consultation about the patients. They certainly do provide a forum for relatives talking to sister, especially, and the social worker about the patients but on the other hand they are cast in fairly general terms so that, if a relative wishes to seek some very specific piece of advice or make some very specific suggestion, they have to do this either by collaring a member of staff before or after the meeting (which they tend not to do, because there really isn't an occasion for this), or, as is more frequent, by interjecting a specific enquiry into the general discussion of the group. This is what happened on this occasion but it's somewhat of a confusion as to whether it really is a discussion about one particularly patient or else a general question about, say, the diets of all the patients in the hospital which may be of interest to other relatives as well. Certainly Miss H did not get a very specific conclusion to her enquiry and was not really in a position to push home the point any further without seeming to introduce an inappropriately personal component to the general discussion.

This field note illustrates, in addition, a dilemma which staff also face. They wish to respond to relatives' requests for advice but, in such an uncertain field as psychogeriatrics, specific advice carries risks and they are most reluctant to stray beyond the immediate bounds of what they see as their area of competence. This field note was based on one of the early meetings of the group and, as time has passed, fairly detailed discussion of individual cases has become somewhat more established as acceptable to both staff and relatives. However, advice still is restricted to comparatively simple and practical aspects of managing the patient and rarely extends to issues of diagnosis, treatment prescription, precise prognosis or the individual allocation of hospital resources, and since staff remain ambivalent about the appropriateness of extended personal discussions, when these do occur they attempt to broaden discussion by drawing out general themes which they consider to be relevant to other relatives. The following example demonstrates the ways in which staff intermix these general points with personal consultations:

> SISTER [explaining one patient's behaviour to their relative]: 'I think the reason he shuts himself into the room when people come in is that he's got a lot of insight into his condition [Mrs D agrees], y'know depressed people know what's going on, and they see the difference in themselves, and he'll not like anyone he knew before to see him as he is now so they tend to shut themselves away; the more they shut themselves away the more depressed they become . . .'

The point is that relatives' consultations are potentially disruptive from a staff point of view because of the opportunity that they provide for relatives to make demands on staff time and services. Used as it is by staff, the relatives' group functions to reduce this problem and also provides a forum for a limited type of individual consultation for a minority of relatives, with minimal impact on the life of the hospital. In addition, by doing this, it functions to maintain amongst staff the notion that individual consultation is widely and readily available to relatives.

Resource allocation

A third function of the group is to convey to relatives a model of the way in which the processes of admission, discharge and patient assessment take place. As the consultant's letters to the GPs frequently comment, patients are admitted initially for 'assessment'. (A decision upon whether they will remain at the hospital is, strictly speaking, taken at six-weekly intervals although – as we have shown in Chapter 6, where we discussed the notion of assessment more fully – in practice matters are not that clear.) Nevertheless staff need to keep the option of discharge open and explain to relatives that the simple fact of having gained a place at the day hospital is not to be read as having obtained permanent access to psychogeriatric services. On the other hand, relatives are clearly disturbed by knowing that there is a decision-point every few weeks which might entail the loss of the place. So staff have a dilemma. While they do not wish to make a firm decision about the patient at an early stage, this reluctance generates uncertainty for relatives. The uncertainty can be contained at the group. The following is an extract from field notes on one group discussion on the issue of discharge:

> Social worker [addressing relative]: 'How do you find . . . [hesitantly] . . . this is the nasty one now . . . about the possibility of the relatives coming home . . . [as if to anticipate the reaction] with the possibility of coming in again?' The atmosphere was tense. One didn't have to be a very skilful observer to get that far. Sister filled the vacuum: 'To give everyone a fair share – and not just twenty-five.' The social worker and sister both explained that: 'There is a six-weekly assessment – everyone is assessed each six weeks.' There was a period of quiet and it was clear what all of the relatives were thinking but Miss N was the first to express it: 'It would not be good for me . . .' The social worker: 'Would it be important to know?' [i.e. that discharge was coming in order to be able to make some arrangements]. Mrs E: 'For us? . . . I think he has improved a bit . . . but I was at the end of my tether before he came here . . . I could not take any more. I thought he would have to be committed.' Miss N: 'Well that is how it was for me . . . that was the alternative for me.' Sister said she well understood this but 'That is O.K. for twenty-five but there are perhaps 3,000 with the same problem – the situation is so chronic – we just give you a break, that is what the day hospital is for.' The social worker: 'But I think we shall make it clear – or else you will get a shock' – [she is explaining that they won't simply be faced with a very sudden announcement of the imminent return of their relative]. Miss N: 'Well I did get a shock – I didn't realize that it was on a six-week basis.' The social worker explained that perhaps the patient would be discharged for a period but might then be taken back after that. Miss N: 'Well you tell us how we can cope in that period – that is it and you tell us . . . I was at the end of my tether.' Miss D [entering the discussion without being prompted]: 'Yes . . . in that period.'

We noted that there had been some change over time in the way in which individual consultation became acceptable within the group. Again, with this third function, there has been some change in emphasis over the period of the group's operation. This has come about as the group has had to adapt to accommodate changes in the day hospital. There has been a trend towards greater severity of condition in the population of patients admitted to the day hospital and those relatives attending the group have generally been coping with patients in more advanced stages of illness. It became increasingly difficult for staff to maintain a model of early discharge from the day hospital in the face of relatives frequently pressing for admission of the patient to a permanent hospital bed. Staff therefore have had to move discussion from the rationing of day hospital places to the process by which in-patient beds are allocated. The following extract is from the transcript of a comparatively recent group meeting:

> SOCIAL WORKER: '... but of course in many cases y'know they are maybe at a stage where they're past that stage ...'
>
> SISTER: '... and we're just trying to give more of the relatives some relief, if the patient is so demented and there's nothing we can do with them, there's an intermediary factor, to give you relatives time to relax, get on with your ordinary lives, give you a break until such time as a bed is available, but the bed situation just now is just terrible. There's nothing, that's why places like the day hospital have grown up, and there's a great need for them.'
>
> SOCIAL WORKER: 'You know what the bed situation is, you'll always hear us saying right along the way, that the bed situation has been bad. We've been going two-and-a-half years now and the bed situation has never been good, never. But it does improve with being able to place people appropriately as we go along, it's improved slightly, and when each one of you, obviously each one of you thinks your own case is impossible, they are impossible. It's not that we deny that, but because we're looking at all of you when we have a bed and we're saying, 'Right we've got a bed', it's the one that's the very worst case at that time, and it doesn't need to be that time, it may be that you've had a long time of waiting – that's taken into account when we're making that assessment, of what person gets the bed. So people are not jumping the gun if you like, just because something terrible has happened today, and they happened to be there at the time and are just at cracking point ...'
>
> SISTER: 'We actually maintain a list in the department of patients who are for long-term care, and if the bed situation got better and we had two or three beds, and there were no crisis or emergencies or people who were so bad then we would try and work down the list. That's if we get a couple of beds but it's very very rarely now because of the set up in the health department just now. That's the way it would work, we always keep a list, a list of short-relief admissions. That's something we could maybe mention as well. [The social worker] mentioned the shared-bed accommodation, which is a step to long-term care, it gives two relatives the relief instead of one relative, or one group of relatives. We try, if we can, if we have a bed at all, short-term admission to give them a break at some point or other to get them away from the stress, and try to keep a list for that as well. Everybody in the department – we put down dates and if there is a bed available at that time then we try and give you the accommodation, if we can, and the social worker can try Part 4 accommodation if the relative's suitable ...'

Staff members who run the group even express some pride in the fact that, because of the work of the group, relatives who attend are extremely unlikely to exert pressure on the hospital in other ways. For example, there is some evidence that group attendance has controlled harassment of the consultant by relatives who are attempting to gain a permanent bed for their patient.

Negotiating the condition

We have already explained that the models which staff and relatives have of the nature of the patient's condition are frequently not one and the same. On the one hand we have indicated that an ideology of active rehabilitation is a central feature of this hospital and this entails the view that the patients have the potential to recover. Most relatives, on the other hand, appear to adopt a view that patients have chronic problems which are likely to deteriorate progressively. The relatives' group serves in its fourth function as a forum for negotiation between these views. The following field note describes one example:

> Sister was explaining that what the hospital hoped to do was to get a particular patient 'to a peak'. Mrs T (the patient's wife): 'Then do they come only for a short period?' Sister said that they were hoping to discharge and then perhaps pick the patients up again and, 'then we can give more people benefit' ... Mrs T: 'But to me – he is making no progress.' Mrs T Junior: 'He's getting worse.' Sister: 'But we get him to shave.' Mrs T: 'Aye but he won't do it with me.' Sister: 'I'll have to give you a uniform', [joking].
>
> There then followed a discussion about uniform and about the decision that they had taken for the staff to wear uniforms in the hospital when it began ...
>
> Mrs T would not be diverted from her insistence that her husband was not in fact improving. Mrs T: 'But he's getting worse with his toilet – does he go by himself here?' Sister [by way of having to react to the relative's production of specific evidence to demonstrate that the patient was not improving at home]: 'But we have a toileting plan – he wouldn't eat at all at first' [produces contrary evidence to counteract the argument about toileting]. Mrs T: 'He will not eat at home and makes a great deal of mess,' [she has previously told stories about what a mess he makes when he eats at home]. 'He said he doesn't get any food here ...' There then followed a set of funny stories about how they found tablets all over the place where Mr. T had hidden them. ... Mrs T begins to sum up her views: 'But if you said he's not here for evermore ... then you can rehabilitate him ... but I say how can you do that ... When he first came here he would be stripped to the waist and washed and shaved (i.e. when the bus came to collect him in the morning) but now I have to do it ...' Sister explains that even if it takes a long time it is better to let the patients dress themselves. Mrs T: 'But now he does dress himself – but after a fashion ...' [Hilarious description of his wearing braces over the top of his jacket and so on].

Therapy for relatives

Fifthly the relatives' group serves to provide what staff describe as a therapy for relatives. Staff, and the social worker in particular, view relatives also as 'clients', if not 'patients' of the institution, and the group as an occasion for providing 'support' to relatives. In particular, staff are offering to relatives opportunities to relieve 'the stress of the burden' by sharing their problems with other group members in a way that they are presumed not to be able to do in other social settings. This is both because the bizarre behaviours of some patients are embarrassing to report in normal company and because those who complain about the burden risk being seen as incompetent carers (Voysey 1975). The following example shows how relatives are themselves clearly seen to be in need of help in coming to acknowledge their problems:

> DAUGHTER 2: 'And of course he just flies at my Mum, he's always taken it off her before but now he's not.' [DAUGHTER 1 simultaneously: 'My mother led the way, and he's no having it any more.']
> SISTER: 'That's the difficulty y'see, because in quite a lot of circumstances the personality completely changes. You get a very quiet person changing into a very aggressive person and your Mum'll try and camouflage that because she remembers what your Dad was like and she wants you to remember him as he was.'
> DAUGHTER 2: 'Exactly.'
> SISTER: '... which leaves her to deal with an awful lot of problems that she could be getting a lot more help from you and she could from us, but until she starts telling us about ...'
> DAUGHTER 2: 'She doesn't want it, this is it.'

Certainly, although relatives may not always define this as a therapy, they undoubtedly do appreciate being able to talk about their troubles with those whom, they feel, share a common experience. They repeatedly engage in what we have come to describe as 'story telling', these sections of the meetings often being accompanied by great hilarity and indeed the stories are frequently very funny in a macabre kind of way. For example:

> Sister then asked Mrs C how her mother was going on with the toilet. Mrs C explained that there was no particular problems but her mother would leave the door open. She then told the story amid a tense mixture of hilarity and gross embarrassment of her mother sitting on the toilet with the door open when her husband and two of his mates had come in the front door.

The tone of the meeting can change from the hilarious to the emotional very rapidly, as shown in this transcript of one relative's story at another group:

> MRS X: 'When I started with him in bed at first when he took his illness, the doctor, and I got a ... the nurse came in and I got a laxative instead of something to firm him up, what a mess I had! Laxative! So I said to the nurse when she came in, I said, "Nurse there's something far wrong," I said, "I got a bottle from the doctor but", I says, "it must have been for the opposite thing" [Lots of laughs]. [The nurse] says, "I think it is," she says, "Aye that's awful, I'll need to let [the doctor] know, I'll go down and tell." [Daughter: 'I don't know how he's still going.'] [The doctor] came in with his head down like that [Demonstrates]. I said "Did you hear about the bottle?" ... and he took the bottle away. A laxative!' [Confused comments, then Mrs X recalls the comments of a friend Mr B].
> MRS X: '... "you're a wee brick, I've never seen anybody had as much work," he said; "it's a good thing you are the nature you are." '
> SISTER: 'You make sure you give him that pellet, he must have that ... O.K.? It is the wee yellow one ...'
> MRS X: 'I've had to work hard all my life, for my mother lived till she was eighty-six and I was there every day, and she was a widow when she was forty-three and I was fifteen and we had, talk about the hardships now and they're

talking about the times we're living in. I mind in the 1920s I was born in 1901, and in the 1920s I had two brothers ... depression and one of the brothers went to the Air Force, because he couldn't get a job. He came on well, he was a warrant-officer when he finished and the other brother died when he was forty-two just because of all the depression, jobs and that [Sister: 'It was a hard time.'] Then ... sister was another tragedy. I've had a lot of troubles myself but not [Sister: 'physical'.] I've managed [Sister: 'But we want to keep you like that'] to cope. Mr B always says "I know you've stood up to it," but I think the harder the struggle the better, you feel you've got the back to it. On Sunday, I was telling you, and I've told ... on Sunday morning I'd given up, I'd never broke down till Sunday morning and that's nearly over a year. On Sunday morning I was doing my potatoes and I just, the services had been on before that, and I just heard somebody say to me, "Fight the good fight with all thy might". It was as clear as that, it wasnae imagination. I had just that put into me, "Oh fight", to fight it, and I tried although I've broken down two or three times this week, just because no having the work to keep me going.'

SISTER: 'You're just getting it all out of your system. I hope you realize now you've got your daughters who are very good, you're no yourself when you're carrying on that fight, you've got everyone in the department here and I'm sure all the relatives here, we're all here to help each other that you've no to keep everything to yourself and try and make a go of it yourself [Mrs W: 'Yes'], and don't hesitate to phone if there's anything, or come up if there's anything, I mean ... because that's no good for you. You end up ill at the end of it all if you keep everything to yourself and try to go it all alone ...'

Relatives do experience very intense emotional reactions because of the stress of coping for long periods with their severely disturbed patients. The relatives' group provides a setting where they feel able, and are encouraged, to express some of the pent-up anger, guilt and distress which they feel. This kind of emotional release is not encouraged at other times or in other areas of hospital life where coping with distressed or irate relatives is viewed by staff as encroaching on their time and disrupting the smooth running of the hospital. Thus although the group does provide a service to relatives in terms of emotional therapy, in so doing it functions as an organizational mechanism for confining that emotion and anxiety to an area where it has little effect on the overall operation of the day hospital.

However, there are limitations to the levels of emotional distress which can be accommodated even within the group and there are occasions when relatives overstep these boundaries. Staff in these instances must find some alternative mode of dealing with the 'trouble' and this is usually achieved by ensuring that such events are handled outside the mainstream of the group meeting. Staff may do this either by confining the interaction of the troublesome relatives to a smaller subgroup in which staff members are the only other participants or, in some cases, by physically isolating the problem by suggesting that the matter should be dealt with separately after the meeting. Sometimes distressed relatives absent themselves from the meeting, on which occasions a member of staff invariably follows them and again counsels them apart from the main group. In this way even extreme distress can be handled without encroachment on the day-to-day work of the hospital.

In these sections of the chapter then, we have been describing the nature of the relatives' group as a part of the day hospital. First we described the group's meetings in general terms. Then we described the functions that it fulfils in coping with relatives while confining them effectively to a limited sector of the institution. During the course of this account the different interests and perspectives of relatives on the one hand and staff on the other have emerged as a significant feature. In the next section we deal more explicitly, on the basis of our interviews data, with the way in which the different constituents of the hospital see the group as affecting their positions.

Constituents' interests

Relatives

First, we deal with the interests of relatives. The relatives have two main objectives in attending the group. They are seeking advice and information about their patient and they value the opportunity of sharing their feelings with other relatives. Relatives who have attended the group expressed their appreciation of it in terms of these objectives when we interviewed them:

> INTERVIEWER: 'You were at the relatives' group there for the first time. What did you think of that?'
> MRS N: 'Oh, I learned an awful lot ... You had no idea what the centre looked like because she [i.e. the patient] would just never ever tell you. That to see the place was a surprise because ... it was lovely – and then to meet the staff was nice.'

> INTERVIEWER: 'You were at the relatives' group there for the first time. What did you think of that?'
> MRS S: 'I quite enjoyed it. It made you feel a wee bit better after you came oot because you felt you werenae on your own. I mean there was quite a few there. Their problems were more difficult than the ones that we're having.'

> INTERVIEWER: 'What did you think about the relatives' support group?'
> MRS H: 'Oh, I enjoyed that. I didn't in the beginning, I thought, "I don't know what I'm doing here, I could be home doing my ironing or something, I don't see that I'm going to learn anything here". But as the night went on you did. And I think there's a lot of therapy in it as well. I think they mean you to unwind, they mean you to open up, they mean you to start talking about your problems, that's half the reason for the support group really. But in a sense, it was, I'll tell you what it was, it provided that, it is useful in the fact that you can unwind, you can talk – here at last is somebody you can talk to and somebody that'll listen to you.'

In these respects the group appears to be providing a very useful service from the relatives' point of view although, in terms of individual consultation, it does have its limitations. As this same group member explained:

> ... I mean at the relatives' support group it is difficult to put over personal things to sister or anybody because there are other relatives sitting there as well and they'll be equally anxious to know about their relative and it would seem as if you were pushing your case too much if you say to sister, 'What did doctor think about my mum, what did he say?'. It is something you would prefer to do in private anyway.

As a general conclusion the functions which we have described on the basis of our own observations accord closely with the terms in which relatives themselves evaluate the usefulness of the group in providing them with a service. The following is a summary of the main points that emerge from our interviews with relatives. They are particularly appreciative of the opportunity which the group provides for finding out about the day hospital and exchanging information about their patient with staff, although they do have reservations about its functioning as a forum for 'personal consultation'. Some relatives feel that this would be more appropriately conducted in a private setting. In any case they would particularly like the chance to have a private discussion with the consultant, which they do not seem to feel they have. Relatives also see the group as a source of information on the processes of 'resource allocation' and as an occasion for putting forward their own particular case for additional help. The possibility exists in the minds of some relatives that by attending the group and providing staff with a full picture of the difficulties at home they might enhance the prospects for a long-term admission. The most frequently cited benefit of group attendance is that of emotional support. Some relatives qualify this point with comments to the effect that attendance may make them feel better in the short term but that this has no effect upon their problems in the long term. The group function which we identified as 'negotiating the condition' does not feature in relatives' evaluation of the group, probably because the processes are subtle and because relatives usually have their own idea about the nature of the patient's condition and are not looking to the group to provide this.

Staff

As we have indicated, the group also fulfils several useful functions for staff. These vary depending upon the different positions which staff members occupy within the hospital.

From the point of view of the nursing staff at the day hospital, the main benefits lie in assisting them in their day-to-day work activities.

> INTERVIEWER: 'What do you see as being the main functions of the relatives' group?'
> SISTER: 'For me, providing support and reducing stress [i.e. among relatives] and I get a lot of information from the relatives about my patients, and as I say that goes into the Kardex. That helps me in planning the total care of the patient. It's O.K. that ... we develop these people and they're not aggressive in the department, they're not incontinent in the department but I'm getting the reports from home that they are totally incontinent and that they're very aggressive and that they're knocking lumps out of this, that and the next person but when you're actually sitting face to face with the relative and the relative is explaining the problem, you know exactly what is going on and it gives you a total picture of your patient rather than just seeing what you see in the department, as I say, which can be the reverse of what they are at home – hm ... the relieving of stress as I say is, and education is, a big part of my role I think in the group to educate the relative to the patient's illness and what we can do about it, the use of medications and the abuse of medications which goes on in homes, in certain homes, educating them there, about that.'

Although the consultant psychiatrist is not actively involved in organizing the group, he too derives direct benefit from it in the performance of his routine duties. The group not only provides an arena in which the relatives' own emotional disturbances can be dealt with but also confronts them with the fact that resources are scarce and that some form of rationing is inevitable. Without the group the consultant would find himself more often having to cope with these problems. He is thus very appreciative of the part played by the group in freeing him of tasks which he would otherwise have to perform. As the consultant that we quoted in Chapter 4 (p. 52) explained:

> Now [the group] seems to have been of great value - hm - in all sorts of ways - hm - like - hm letting people know that there is a big problem in the shortage of accommodation because they hear other people and see other people with the same sort of problems, but that's maybe not even the most important thing, it provides a setting where people can abreact, they can talk about their feelings and embarrassment and aggression in a group of people who are all on the same footing and I think this is very valuable ... I'm now sometimes going into a situation in somebody's home where the main problem really is, say, the daughter's feelings about her dementing mother or father where I almost feel that they don't really need to take the patient on but I'd like to take the relatives.

The social worker, as the member of staff with most involvement with the problems of the patients' families, might be expected to have the greatest commitment to the concept of a support group for relatives. Certainly, for her, it is an economical means of providing the relatives with the type of service that is otherwise, in a medical setting, likely to be lacking. The social worker made the point:

> Support is - hm - you've got people who come [to the group] who are really isolated. All the things about communication and isolation that I was talking about earlier. They are the people that are lost. You've got someone who's confused and who is needing help which you can deal with here - hm - you can't deal with that, with these people out there, on a one-to-one kind of thing - hm - not all the time anyway. Hm - and the doctor doesn't do that. He doesn't give them the kind of thing that they understand and the empathy or whatever that is required. So that's the support. Adding on to that kind of support, you have things like enquiries. 'What do I do if mother jumps up in the middle of the night and streaks about the flat?' Hm - now sister can answer quite a lot of those kind of things. That's support. Somebody else tells you that that their mother has done this. There's not a relative yet, I think, really who has ever said to another relative, 'I am worse than you'. I don't think they've ever said that but what they've done is talk about themselves and the other relatives think 'They're worse than me'.

Thus, although nurses, consultant and social worker have somewhat different interests in the group they are not mutually incompatible. (There *is* a good deal of incompatibility on some matters between staff interests and those of relatives, as we have noted, but these different perspectives seldom emerge as open conflict. There are several reasons for this. Staff present an image of the group as consistent with an overall hospital aim of service to relatives. Relatives are encouraged to believe that the group is their own group yet in practice staff control the patterns of social interactions in the group.)

This is not to imply that the history of the group has been without conflict between members of staff. In the early stages of its development there was by no means complete consensus about its purposes. As we noted earlier, administrative staff saw the initial idea as alien to the traditional picture of a hospital in which there are clear boundaries between the institution and the patient's home. While the social worker saw such a group as central to the day hospital's innovative programme, nursing administrators were inclined to view it as a diversion of resources away from patient care. The nursing staff were in an ambiguous position, with loyalty to their senior officers but also with considerable sympathy for the views of colleagues from other disciplines, with whom they saw themselves working in new relationships within a novel kind of service.

We have already mentioned the particular points on which there was disagreement. Generally, the conflict which arose centred around the degree of control which hospital administrative staff could exert over the activities of the group and was eventually, at least for most practical purposes, resolved by their acceptance of indirect monitoring through the usual nursing hierarchy. Although senior staff have remained somewhat uneasy about this resolution, particularly about the possibility of loss of control in the event of staff changes, most conflict was short-lived and has occasioned no significant disruption to the organization or activities of the group. Staff who are not directly involved with the group now respond to its work with acceptance or mild indifference. Indeed the acceptance has been possible because the group does not hinder them in *their* day-to-day work. So all staff may value the relatives' group as an expression of service to relatives, and this as one basis for describing the success of the hospital as a whole, for reasons which in specific terms vary but which nevertheless are presented as being in general accord.

This is in sharp contrast to the way in which other criteria for evaluating the success of the hospital are operationalized. For example, in describing the ways in which different groups of staff perceive and pursue 'patient flow' as a goal (in Chapter 5) we noted not only that what counts as a desirable pattern of patient admission and discharge differs between staff depending upon their organizational locale, but also that the activities designed to foster such a pattern are inclined to generate 'trouble' for staff whose interests vary because of the organizational position which they occupy. The activities of admission and discharge have very direct practical implications for all staff. So conflict amongst staff basically reflects self-interest. In the case of the relatives' group however, as we have indicated, some staff express reservations but without any great fervour because in their own work they can remain largely immune from its activities. The reason for this is that, unlike admission and discharge, the involvement of relatives is not central to the main work of the hopsital. Quite the contrary. Since relatives' issues are organizationally isolated within the relatives' group, staff can support the group in terms which vary but which do not complicate the work of other staff. On the other hand, staff who do not value it may express this as indifference, rather than as practical limitation or outright opposition.

Conclusion

Our analysis in this chapter of a relatives' group in a psychogeriatric day hospital contrasts with other research literature dealing specifically with support groups for relatives of the elderly mentally infirm. This literature is largely confined to describing the themes which emerge in group discussions and the benefits which relatives derive from attendance.

Barnes et al. (1981) and Lazarus et al. (1981) describe the use of time-limited groups with relatives of Alzheimer patients. In both cases the group was set up as a result of clinicians' awareness of the problems experienced by relatives of patients and in the knowledge that similar groups had proved useful in dealing with the families of aphasic and stroke patients. Fuller et al. (1979) report on the formation, again on the initiative of clinicians, of support groups for the relatives of dementia patients. These groups approximate more closely to that which we have described in this book. Unlike the Alzheimer groups, they run continuously with a changing membership. Though catering essentially for relatives of patients with some form of dementia, they also include relatives of some patients with functional disorders.

In these three studies the central themes identified in the group discussions are very similar, variations probably being attributable to differences in the context and operation of the groups. These themes include lack of understanding and knowledge about the illness, lack of support and information from the health professions, problems in coping with patients' behaviour, emotional reactions to the patients, feelings of isolation and loss of self-identity.

The emphasis throughout these studies is on the effect of the group on the individual relatives' adjustment to their situation. Fuller is alone in noting that staff may also gain from involvement in the groups. This, he suggests, occurs through the acquisition of increased information and insight into the problems of caring for the dementia patient. However, although they are not discussed explicitly in terms of the successfulness of the groups, Fuller, in outlining the rationale for the formation of groups, also alludes to other group functions not directly concerned with benefit to relatives. The groups described by Fuller were set up in an area of shortage of in-patient resources, and where some relatives cared for patients ar home for longer than was desirable. This resulted in pressure on doctors in the form of relatives contacting them to say that they could no longer cope with the patient. The doctor was required to spend time with relatives discussing their problems until they reached the stage of 'returning home with the problem unchanged but apparently satisfied and willing to carry on caring for their elderly relatives'. The group setting enabled this kind of ventiliation and support to be carried out in a manner which was economic in terms of professional time. In general however, by concentrating on individual patients and relatives and neglecting the organizational context of the groups, these studies imply that groups function only to assist relatives and neglect those broader consequences for the hospital system which, so far as we can judge from our own research, may be equally significant.

So, in this chapter our approach has been to treat the study of a relatives' group as part of our wider study of the services of a new psychogeriatric day hospital. We began by recalling how service to relatives is widely advanced within the hospital as one important evaluative criterion. The relatives' group has been developed in pursuit of 'success' in these terms. Yet, as we have indicated, relatives do not in practice impinge as systematically on major areas of hospital life as the widespread advocacy of an ideology of service to relatives, extending beyond relief by mere custodial care of the patient, would lead us to expect. For example, some relatives do visit the hospital but the majority do not; some, but by no means all, have contact with the nursing auxiliaries who escort the patients on the bus to and from the hospital but this contact is fleeting and with low-status staff; relatives are often seen by the psychiatrist on his initial domiciliary visit but play no direct part in the negotiations over admission and generally there is no further contact with the psychiatrist to discuss his reasons for discharge; some relatives do have contact with a social worker for assessment prior to patient admission but routine subsequent contact is largely with relatives of patients likely to occasion a 'crisis' for the hospital; relatives can request an appointment with the consultant but seldom do; staff do say that relatives are welcome to participate in the daily social activities of the hospital but in practice this is extremely rare; there is no systematic and routine mechanism for exchanging information about the day-to-day life of the patient in the hospital and at home. Throughout this chapter we have described how the relatives' group fulfils a number of useful functions in terms of providing service to relatives. These might otherwise have been fulfilled in other ways. In effect the group has served to provide some additional contacts with relatives but in a way which isolates them from the day-to-day life of the hospital and so reduces any threat to the smooth running of hospital routines. Moreover, staff and administrators are able to feel that the hospital is organized in accord with the ideology of service to relatives because of the existence of such a group.

We have described the events at group meetings in some detail and listed the main categories of interaction as exchange of information, individual consultation, resource allocation, negotiating the condition, and thereapy for relatives. We have shown how both staff and relatives benefit from this interaction but how, in areas of differing interests, staff retain control. We have also outlined the different staff interests in the group and have suggested that, in spite of some initial conflict, and in spite of the different interests, the group has nevertheless attracted general support. The reason for this is that relatives' issues have not been systematically and organizationally incorporated into the hospital and thus do not generally complicate the day-to-day work of staff. Indeed, to return to the thesis with which we began this chapter, the group maintains an ideology of service to relatives (and presents a successful image of the hospital on this criterion) but effectively limits its practical implementation to a self-contained and rather isolated locale which minimizes the problems of 'relative disturbance' to the organization overall.

CHAPTER ELEVEN

Success as Quality of Service

Introduction

Through earlier chapters we have been explaining that there are a variety of criteria of success in terms of which the performance of the day hospital is evaluated. Although this performance is variable, we have noted that on each criterion there is a very distinct sense of achievement within the culture of the hospital. At various points in the study we have described how this 'ideology of success' is maintained.

Yet, in spite of the widespread and very strong 'culture of achievement', it would be wrong to imply that professional staff and administrators do not on occasions themselves have doubts about the effective operation of the hospital. After all, many staff can make many of the observations that we have been able to make and are in a position to conclude that the available information does not on all occasions justify the view of success which participants promote – although it is true that few people within the organization are in a position to view it from the variety of perspectives which we have been able to adopt. Some staff, at least, are very much aware, for example, that the ability of the hospital to offer a clinical cure to some groups of patients is limited; that although the hospital has not 'silted up' aspects of patient flow are far from ideal; that the services which the hospital offers are not as well integrated as they might be; and so on. Nevertheless, as we have observed, the notion that the day hospital is successful has proved to be remarkably resilient over a considerable period of time. In this chapter we suggest that this occurs because, failing all else, staff can fall back on 'commonsense' notions about satisfactory care of the elderly. These include positive attitudes amongst staff, the comfort and cleanliness of the building, the quality of meals, the patients' happiness, enjoyment of activities, and so on. Amongst staff there is a more or less shared view about what constitutes 'civilized' and 'kindly' treatment of the elderly mentally infirm. Pictures of the grosser deficiencies of large, old and understaffed institutions for the elderly are common to many of those engaged in planning and providing the service and there is a widespread feeling that this new day hospital is at least rather more successful than them in providing a comfortable, humane and decent environment.

Against this background it is not surprising that, as we outlined in Chapter 4, one major criterion for judging the success of the hospital refers to the *quality* of the service. In this chapter we shall outline the ways in which staff describe and fall back upon this criterion. They highlight those aspects of hospital life, the impact of which may be hard to measure in any very specific way but which nevertheless are seen as extremely important in contributing to the general impression of a high-quality environment. These features are regarded as valuable in their own right rather than in any particular instrumental way. Then, in the second part of this chapter, we shall present some evidence on the ways in which relatives view the quality of the service which their patients receive.

Quality of service

Staff views

Firstly, staff point to the quality of the physical environment. As we have described, the day hospital is a purpose-built structure and well furnished. Many staff commented upon this fact, for example:

> I think that having a reasonable building does help, and very few day hospitals are as nice as this. I suppose you have noticed having been round other ones. They often used discarded accommodation in various places, sometimes a ward, sometimes its been also a gym, or something like this, an old sitting-room or something, whereas this was built as a day hospital, it's not an also ... an also-ran.
>
> (*A nursing officer*)

Indeed, arguments in support of a high standard of physical provision had been advanced from the earliest stages of planning the hospital, the justification being that it would improve the quality of life for the patients. One member of staff described the impact of the resultant comfortable, well equipped environment:

> [The planner] said, 'If you put a good carpet down people will not wet it.' They don't. If you put lino down they'll wet it. They don't do as they're told. Do as you want them to, you see. So he fought very hard to get top quality carpet and if they put lino and they wet it it was easier to clean up but the patients are aware that it is a very good carpet and they don't want to wet it, so they don't ... well, you know ... aim to try and stop people so I really feel that many – the mirror, full-length mirror for example, for dressing, the fact that there's a bed and its not a hospital bed, there's only one bed and the ... the standard of ... the fact that the patients sometimes help clean up the dishes and things, the fact that the television isn't on all the time, its only on when people want to see something they particularly want to see. The fact that I've looked in through the windows when its been dark then all the patients are all interested in what they're doing. They might

be resting but they are interested in it, they're not actually, you know, as they often are with their coats on waiting to go away, they're interested in what's going on and they've obviously either been active or quite happy with what they are doing and they don't have to be knitting or anything as long as they are just ... they're very much human beings when they're there, which I think is very important. Many day hospitals are in fact ... [the patients are] zombies. Just another place to sit and a bit of different company but not very much else.

(*Community medicine specialist*)

During the early years, the hospital's high standards continued to be afforded a degree of protection by the health board, which took the view that having launched this initiative it was only sensible to allocate to it sufficient resources to allow it to prove its worth, although, as one health board official explained, this policy was not without its critics:

Well the thing that impressed me about the day hospital is the standard of finish because - hm - although I've been in purpose-built day hospitals before in England - hm - I wasn't very impressed by the high standard of finish. I'm not quite clear in my own mind as to whether that high standard of finish was necessary; we have been very criticized for it, you know, there are a lot of people who have said 'Well, we [could] have had two for the price of one'; if we hadn't gone for such ... its a very attractive building to go into it. It's a very stimulating building.

Nevertheless in several aspects of its services the hospital retained a relatively high level of resource input. For example, in transport arrangements for patients a bus contract was allowed in preference to the use of the ambulance service. Also the arrangements for using nurses to accompany patients during the bus journey is expensive in staff time but nevertheless justified as improving the quality of patient care. As an administrator explained:

... the idea of an old lady jumping on a No. 1 bus and trotting along to the day hospital just doesn't work in the care of psychogeriatric patients, they need to be escorted there, they need to be carefully looked after and of course in the case of the day hospital the nurse goes in with them when they get home and so on, we feel that is very essential and therefore there is a *high* transport cost and a *high staff input*.

A favourable 'quality of life' springs from staff attitudes as well as from the physical environment. The social worker made this point as follows:

INTERVIEWER: 'When patients are actually here during the day, what sort of things do you think are happening that they are benefiting from that are helping towards improving ...'
SOCIAL WORKER: 'The quality of life ... I think that one ... I think the *main* thing that happens here is the warmth of the place. I think that there's a very very strong - correct me if I'm wrong but I think there' s a very strong warm feeling in here which I think gets through to the very confused - again as I say you can go into a ward, or I could take you to Part 4 [local authority accommodation] and I could take you to where people *care*. There's a word, care, because they look after them and protect them sort of thing, but there is no warm feeling, in fact there is quite a *horrible* sometimes when you go in. That doesn't happen here and perhaps the structure of the building helps, you know, that it's pretty open plan ...'

It is seen as essential that staff do not adopt commonly held stereotypes of the elderly mentally infirm but get to know their patients' personalities and respond to their individual needs.

> I get very annoyed at times - eh - at how people are apt to look at psychogeriatric or confused old people that they have no further to go and its only a matter of looking at them and looking after them I should say and caring for them and that's *it* - I don't believe that - I think that you can improve the quality of life for anyone and no matter how confused they are I think there's a spark ... the caring is not always the physical looking after, the caring is trying to find out what an individual is trying to tell you or what they require and *that* to me is where the caring comes in, because if you can recognize that, *then* you can care enough to help them to get it...
>
> (*A social worker*)

Such an approach to patient care ensures that the hospital provides a stimulating environment which is not only important as an aid to the clinical improvement of the patients but is to be valued in its own right. As a nurse explained:

> It certainly helps them to fill their day. It quite often discovers previous hobbies, pastimes, and stimulates them that way. It may well make them feel more useful again because they are actually doing something at their handicraft session. It depends on the degree of dementia as well, though, but it certainly helps to stimulate them, where if they were at home they might not be stimulated into any of these activities.

So positive attitudes on the part of staff are widely seen as characterizing the day hospital throughout. They are much valued as part of its services and were attributed by our respondents to both the character of individual staff members and adequate staffing levels. Although in the early years of the hospital, as we have described, there was some difficulty in filling all the established posts, generally the day hospital is well staffed by the standards of comparable institutions.

Apart from the high calibre of staff, adequate staffing levels and positive attitudes, our respondents also saw staff morale as being important in the quality of service provision. Certainly senior nursing staff see it as a major part of their job to maintain high staff morale as a component of the quality of care within the hospital:

> ... whereas in this department your job is the patient, my first job is the patient, then my job is the nursing staff, I must keep my nursing staff's morale up, if I don't keep these girls' morale up and keep their interest going in the job, they're going to reflect back on my patients and they're not going to do what we should be doing for the patients...
>
> (*A nursing sister*)

The fact that the majority of staff applied for their posts under some competition and were keen to work in the new hospital in their specific roles was quoted as an important component in the enthusiasm which staff displayed for their work. One administrator who praised the whole atmosphere of the hospital, and remarked on its apparent efficiency and friendliness, saw the style of management and the maintenance of morale as especially important:

> ... the work there is being done in a stimulating environment - you would hardly call, you know, the sort of clinical leadership as being very dominating, there's very much of a team spirit operating, but albeit within the constraints that the team - that your research group has already described - I think there is a lot *going* for the day hospital ...

Relatives' views

Relatives are generally impressed by the hospital's pleasant and comfortable environment and the high standard of care from staff. Most relatives base their comments on either the patients' reaction to attendance or their own limited contact with the institution and they are frequently pleasantly surprised at the conclusions that they draw. In part this surprise stems from the generally low expectation generally which they have of services for the elderly but it is also related to the association which, as we mentioned in Chapter 2, Park Hospital has with the old Poor Law.

In the views of relatives the quality of care has several facets. First they like the building and its furnishings. The daughter of one patient described her initial reaction to the hospital:

> INTERVIEWER: 'What did you think of the day hospital itself?'
> MRS N: 'It is very nice and comfortable, it really is. I was amazed the first time I saw it, I mean I expected a sort of bare - I don't know - an institution thing and it was really completely different from what I thought it would be. I was really amazed when I saw it, I mean there is everything there for their comfort, some of them will be more comfortable than in their own home I am sure, they are bound to be.'

Second, relatives are very appreciative of staff attitudes:

> MR C: 'As far as my own personal judgement about the day hospital, I think it is perfect, and I am quite sure those who fulfil their duty at the day hospital are doing their duty in an exceptional way that one appreciates, I don't feel for any minute that they are not fulfilling their duty or they should be doing more to my wife than they are doing, I have never come out with that in my mind, always leave thankful for any kindness and love that is extended to her when she is there and I appreciate that so much and I know the daughters feel the same.'

Third, relatives are impressed by the way in which the hospital creates a stimulating environment and keeps the patient active and involved. For example:

> INTERVIEWER: 'Has the day hospital done anything to help her this time do you think?'
> MR Z: 'Oh, it does help her, aye. It keeps her active and gies her an interest in things, y'ken. They're always making things, sometimes its dolls, sometims it wee wicker baskets and things like this, crocheting, it always kind of keeps her active and her mind active although she is no terribly fit, it always keps her mind on something.'

Although, as we have already mentioned, many relatives do not have high expectations that the hospital will 'cure' their patient, some of them still expect the patient to derive some benefit from the increased stimulation. For example:

> INTERVIEWER: 'What kind of help did you see the day hospital offering?'
> MISS T: 'Well she'd have company, she'd have things to do, whatever they do down there, I suppose its much the same as [another hospital], making bunnies and all the rest of it. [Laughs.] Gives her some interest apart from wandering the streets.'
> INTERVIEWER: 'Did you think the day hospital would actually be able to offer any specific treatment? To help her condition?'
> MISS T: 'No.'

Fourth, relatives also attach considerable importance simply to whether or not the patient is happy in attending. One relative described with pleasure how her father responds to the prospect of his visits:

> What like was he on Tuesday! See when the bus came up he says, 'Right girls, come, move', and he was down that stair like a two-year-old, he was like a wean goin' on a Sunday school trip. He comes in and he'll say, 'They are great to you out there, they are that nice, nice lassies out there.' [Laughing.]

Another had a similar reaction:

> INTERVIEWER: 'What do you think is the main benefit from her going?'
> MR X: 'I think in herself she's quite happy. They're all very nice to her. You know by what you – there's nobody has told me anything, you're just trying to get – you don't get very much out of her, you see, its only as you keep letting her talk. You see. "Are they nice to you then?" "Oh! aye!" she says, "they're lovely to me. They're lovely they all come round", she says "and they admired my skirt" or jersey or things like that. She's quite tickled.'

However, in spite of this general approval some relatives feel that some patients have deteriorated to such an extent that they cannot fully appreciate the care that they are receiving. They feel that only those patients who are relatively less confused will derive much pleasure and benefit from the hospital:

> Oh! its a lovely place. I am quite sure, it is a pity, maybe they are, it's different if you saw the group, the patients like as a whole, I just imagine they would all be like my Mum, very mentally confused or deteriorating and all the rest of it and don't appreciate, I'm sure she doesn't. I am sure she doesn't know she is going to a nice day centre where she could meet other people and if she could cast her mind back that it's rather like the Women's Guild she used to go to and they give her wee things to do and it could be great. It would be great for people who are compus mentis and yet could fully appreciate that, it would be absolutely super . . . but it is a pity that she can't appreciate that.

Other relatives have some other reservations about the quality of care. First, relatives of patients who are suffering from depression or who are much less confused than the majority of dementia patients often complain that their patients find it disturbing to spend so much time in the company of others who are severely confused. The son of one demented patient said that his mother had complained about the other people at the day hospital and obviously did not see herself as being like them. She had described the hospital as being 'like play-school. You go and get given different things to do and there is a sing-song'.

Second, some relatives complained that patient enjoyment is limited by their having to travel outside their local community to attend the hospital. Their patients are therefore not mixing with people whom they have known over the years.

Finally, although, as we have mentioned, the association of Park Hospital with the Poor Law is not, apparently, important to relatives themselves, many felt that the reputation and stigma associated with this institution remains significant in the mind of the patient.

> MRS H: 'Y'know but to understand, my mother at that age to her Park was – eh – that's whit they ca'd the 'Pairs Hoose', y'know its got that stigma, although its a' different but this is what an awfu' lot of the old folks think, it's the Pairs Hoose, and they havenae a clue, they havenae an idea what like places or how they run or how no. They think its a – shame or somethin' to get in.'

And another relative described an even stronger reaction from the patient:

> MR M: 'One morning ... "where's my caird?" So I says, "There's your caird there" – Its beautiful the day hospital you know – but she reads it and says, "That's the Poores House, your sending me to the Poor House" – oh! what a cairry on I had that morning, her mind's no all that far gone, she's minding when it used to be the old Poor House y'know.'

Conclusion

In this chapter we have set out a final criterion for measuring the success of the day hospital. We have described the way in which staff value the quality of care as a significant achievement of the hospital services. We have shown that amongst relatives there is also widespread agreement that the day hospital provides a pleasant, comfortable and stimulating environment for the patient. Most relatives consider it to be particularly important that the patient should find the experience of attendance an enjoyable one. Despite the reservations which we have noted, there are comparatively few (and then only rather specific) criticisms of the quality of care in these terms.

Undoubtedly, physically the hospital is a pleasant environment in which the elderly can spend the day. The hospital has commanded more than its fair share of resources. The activities are stimulating and well staffed and staff morale is high. Staff are in consequence polite to patients, treat them civilly, and are positively warm in their attitudes towards them.

Some of the objectives for the hospital which we have discussed in other chapters are ambitious and staff are well aware of the constant potential for failure. Yet, as we have shown, a culture of success is essential to the institution's functioning. The criterion of quality of care serves, if all else fails, to maintain the view that in whatever other ways the hospital might be deficient, it cannot be accused of failing in the quality of its attempts.

CHAPTER TWELVE

Summary and Conclusion: Pluralistic Evaluation

Starting-point

We began this book by pursuing a line of argument which, in summary, has run as follows. The issue of evaluation is central to research on health and welfare services but the conventional and predominant mode of evaluative research – essentially experimental, rationalist and objectivist in approach – is fraught with difficulties.

First, there are practical difficulties. When setting up evaluative studies we discover that the controls of the clinical trial are very seldom available. Frequently, also, the nature of the programme that is to be evaluated is unestablished at the start of the investigation and, anyway, typically it changes quite rapidly over time. This is especially true if, as is often the case with evaluative research, it is a novel programme. Thus the evaluators face the problem of having to say that a programme does or does not 'work' without being able to say what the programme is. Furthermore, since, frequently, it is not easy to locate any clear statement of the objective of a new programme and since there are variable views from different groups about what constitutes 'success' in the programme's achievements, the evaluator has the problem of defining and selecting a criterion for evaluation.

These practical difficulties are rooted in theoretical difficulties. For the conventional approach to evaluation makes three very important presumptions. These are the presumption of rationality in the social policy process, the presumption of the experimentalist ideal in social research and the presumption of consensus in professional organizations. All three are unjustified. Serious weaknesses are therefore endemic to the conventional approach and thus the time is ripe to look for new directions in the methodology of evaluative research.

Several suggestions have recently been made about the new directions that this kind of research might take. These include 'process evaluation', 'illuminative evaluation' and exploring the implications for evaluative methodology of subjectivist epistemology and of political and methodological pluralism. Taken together, these suggestions point to a new approach which we have termed pluralistic evaluation. The bulk of the book has been a report on a research project which we have set out as a model for the way in which pluralistic evaluation may proceed.

Now therefore we shall recall the main features of pluralistic evaluation before summarizing the principal findings from our research. We shall then point to the advantages of a pluralistic approach. We are far from complacent, however, about the progress which has been made, and so we conclude with a postscript listing some outstanding issues. Throughout this final chapter we bear in mind that, from the start, our project has adopted a dual focus. By examining the way in which one hospital is functioning we have sought to contribute to an understanding of the operation and development of psychogeriatric services. Through this description the research has also aimed to explore the problems of embarking on evaluations in the field of health and social services.

Features of a pluralistic evaluation

Drawing, then, upon the several strands of the various suggestions that have been made for a 'new approach' to evaluative research we can set out the main features of what we have termed 'pluralistic evaluation'.

(1) As a general feature, the approach is heavily informed by models of institutional functioning and the policy process which draw upon theories of political pluralism. Thus we are sensitized to the importance of varied group interests and power bases and the ways in which the plurality of interests interact in a system of checks and balances upon which the workings of the service are eventually based. This does not exclude an analysis of conflict as between two major (class) groups. But typically in the field of health and welfare services the constituent parties are more numerous than that. It is unlikely that there will be a simple division between 'professionals' on the one hand and 'consumers' on the other. The approach is also heavily influenced by the 'subjectivist' stance within sociology. Thus we are sensitized to the importance of understanding the interpretations which professionals, planners, administrators, relatives and patients place upon the operation of the agencies of which they are a part.
(2) The research must identify the major constituent groups to the policy initiative and, throughout the research, compare them with each other, both in the ideological perspectives that they hold, and in their operational strategies.
(3) In particular, we must collect data on these groups' interpretations and perceptions of 'success' in service provision and assign to that data a central place in the evaluative analysis.
(4) The study must document not only the plurality of notions of success but also the different groups' strategies as they strive to implement their own per-

spectives in their own interests. We take the view that an attempt to disentangle the meanings and pursuit of 'success' is an intrinsic part of the evaluation exercise.

(5) Evaluative research must then assess the extent to which success (or failure) is achieved on each of the several criteria employed within the agency and in terms of the several meanings assigned to these criteria. Success is a pluralistic notion. It is not a unitary measure.

(6) In consequence, pluralistic evaluation must embody the principles of methodological triangulation. It is now widely accepted that any study dependent upon a single data source is 'method-bound'. The point of particular relevance to evaluation research is that each data source tends to be interest-bound (as tied to the interests of one group rather more than to the interests of another) and also ideology-bound (as reflecting one group's perspectives on desirable modes of operation and 'success' rather more than the perspectives of other groups). The constant use of as many different kinds of data as possible ensures, as far as possible, that the research reflects the full range of interests, ideologies, interpretations and achievements abroad within the agency.

(7) Thus pluralistic evaluation offers an ethnography of the way the services function and an explanation of the processes involved (in terms of the pluralistic interests of participating groups) as well as (somewhat complex) conclusions about the success of the services on a range of criteria.

In practice, we should not pretend that it has always been easy to conform to these tenets. We believe, however, that the attempt is rewarding and productive of data that is rich for both explanatory and evaluative purposes. We have also argued that pluralistic evaluation goes some considerable way towards solving the difficulties that we encountered as we embarked upon this research.

In the next section we bring together the conclusions of our study as we examine the performance of the day hospital on several criteria, in line with this approach.

Performance and success

In the early part of our study we identified in Chapter 4 six criteria, advanced by members of the institution, for assessing the 'success' of the day hospital's services. In examining the work of the hospital on each count, much detail emerged which, cumulatively, displayed characteristics of the hospital that are important in relation to evaluative questions.

On the first criterion, that of patient flow, the day hospital has undoubtedly avoided the 'silt up' that characterizes many institutions of this kind. Referrals, which are mainly from GPs, are not always actively promoted. However, patients who are referred are comparatively seldom refused admission. At the end of a year treatment has ceased for about 70% of the patients admitted during that year. Over 60% of discharges are due to a deterioration in the patients' condition and some 20% of discharges occur because the patient and/or relative refuses to allow the patient to continue to attend. A small proportion of patients are discharged to local authority accommodation. By far the largest group of discharges consists of patients who move to an in-patient bed, either permanently or on some short-term or shared arrangement. The hospital is doing little to divert patients from the ultimate destination of in-patient care. Over 20% of patients are offered the facility of a short-term bed and over 30% of day hospital patients progress to a long-term bed. In practice the day hospital is not, however, playing any major role as a stepping-stone in the opposite direction; that is for the outward movement of patients from hospital and into the community.

On the second criterion, that of clinical cure, we conclude that, to judge from the evidence of hospital records, and to judge from the way in which decisions are made in hospital meetings, the success of the hospital is rather limited. This conclusion is supported by a detailed inspection of the files of discharged cases, especially those in which 'discharge back to the community' is equated with 'improvement'. Frequently, no very precise or widely accepted definition of patients' problems serves as a starting-point for their clinical career through the hospital, and insofar as nursing rating scales are indicative of condition, then the majority of patients show very little improvement during their stay at the hospital. At best, the active therapeutic regime of the hospital is having a significant effect on 6% of the cases admitted. A more pessimistic, but well supported conclusion is that hard evidence on clinical improvement is available for an even smaller proportion of the patients who leave the hospital. On the evidence which the hospital itself marshals about its own services, hospital practice cannot be described as the successful pursuit of clinical cure. Even in the small numbers of cases in which the patient is assessed by the hospital staff as having improved, there is apparently little quantifiable data on which these judgements are based. Indeed, decisions are seldom taken on the basis of quantified information about the changes in the patient's condition and in practice the hospital accumulates little specific information, on the patient's progress towards a 'cure', which is actually used in determining the patient's career path.

On the third criterion, the provision of an integrated service, the attempt to provide a range of psychogeriatric and related services through a team of professional staff within the hospital has the following consequences. The division of labour within the team tends to confirm the boundaries between existing specialisms. Social work services are incorporated into the work of the hospital but without disturbing the usual professional hierarchies of medical practice. The day hospital has not really solved the problem of providing a co-ordinated social work/psychiatric service to patients since, even when the services provided by the hospital are effectively co-ordinated, crucial issues remain concerning the co-ordination of hospital services with those provided by outside agencies. The most significant development in integrated resource use – the use of in-patient beds in Park Hospital in close conjunction with day hospital places – has taken place outside the day hospital team. The major problem of co-ordinating day hospital services and the provision of general practice has not been significantly affected by the organization of day hospital services.

The fourth criterion of success is the impact of the day hospital on related services. Our general conclusion is that relationships between the day hospital and related services vary considerably. Our materials are in some instances consistent with the view that it is contributing to the effectiveness of other services. In other instances we are forced to be a little more sceptical.

More specifically, it is undoubtedly important that the day hospital is offering 'relief' to GPs. There are many examples of problems which would continue to be primarily the responsibility of GPs were it not for the hospital's services. Nevertheless not all GP referrals are accepted. Nor are GPs fully relieved of responsibility for those of their patients who do attend the hospital.

Through the social worker attached to the day hospital, the hospital undertakes a good deal of work which can legitimately be described as a social work service. Most of this is in the form of background reports on relatives and other matters geared to the organization and concerns of the hospital. However the day hospital also makes demands upon residential social work services in discharging patients to this form of accommodation. But the numbers involved are very small. Also, since the social worker is primarily concerned only with those aspects of the case which have a bearing upon the patient's attendance at the day hospital, a field worker in an area team must also remain in contact with a case if that case is already known to the social work department.

The day hospital has also made very little difference to the comparatively rigid boundaries which exist between the geriatric and the psychogeriatric systems of care. On the other hand the relationship between the day hospital and the home-help service is a very good example of the way in which resources may effectively be used and, we suspect, net levels of service provision increased. The quality of the relationship between these services contrasts with the quality of relationship between the day hospital and either the geriatric or other social work services.

The question of whether or not the hospital has contributed to the rest of the psychiatric sector of which it is part turns on the issue of whether the day hospital has successfully increased the flow of patients through those parts of this sector which were previously blocked. As we have described, it is a major achievement that patients are moved in and out of the day hospital itself. An additional source of help is thus provided for the excessive number of cases which are referred to the psychiatrists.

On the criterion of providing support to the patients' relatives, the custodial care of patients which the hospital provides is most valuable. It does not ease the problem for relatives at night, when the patient is physically very unwell, when attendance for more than the allocated days is required, or when the costs to relatives of patient attendance outweigh the benefits. To judge from our data, systematic communication between the patient's family and the hospital, emotional support for the relatives and advice on patient care are not very successful aspects of the provision of a service to relatives. The relatives' group does provide one forum for the exchange of information between relatives and staff and provides some relatives with a degree of emotional support but, generally, the group isolates relatives from the main body of the hospital and even further isolates relatives who are unable or unwilling to attend meetings of the group.

Most relatives do not visit the hospital or participate in social activities. They have (fleeting) contact only with nursing auxiliaries, play no direct part in the decisions about patient admission or discharge, do not request an appointment to see the consultant, and do not provide the hospital with regular information about the patient at home. The hospital focuses its main efforts on the individual patient rather than on resolving family difficulties. Consequently the hospital has little impact on the 'problem' as this is construed by relatives.

Finally there is the criterion of quality of service. Undoubtedly there are many features of the hospital's environment which are valuable in their own right and quite apart from their impact in any particular instrumental way. Clearly, the hospital is generally a 'nice place to be'. Physically it offers pleasant surroundings in which the elderly can spend the day, the activities are stimulating, the hospital is well staffed and staff morale is high. Staff are in consequence polite to patients, treat them civilly and are positive in their attitudes towards them. The day hospital provides a pleasant, comfortable and stimulating environment for the patients. Our account of the hospital, its facilities and its staff largely supports the view that in whatever other ways the hospital might fail, it cannot be accused of failing in the quality of its attempt.

Group interests and success

We have said that these statements about performance and success in the hospital are relevant to an evaluative analysis. They do not, however, *constitute* an evaluation. Statements about performance are inadequate in isolation because there are differing views about their significance and meaning. We have identified several criteria of success and we have grouped our conclusions round these themes. But this does not entirely solve the key problem of defining criteria in evaluative research for, as we have shown throughout the study, on each separate criterion there still remains disagreement as to what counts as success. For example, 'cure' may be equated with 'discharge' by hospital staff whereas relatives do not see it that way. High patient turnover in which referrals are accepted and beds are obtained is success for GPs but not for nurses in in-patient wards for whom successful patient flow means the discharge of long-term patients to community (including GP) care. So if we are to decide upon the significance of statements about performance, they must be related not only to statements about the meanings of success but also to statements about the ways in which these meanings are operationalized by the various and vested interest groups involved.

For the picture of the day hospital that has emerged throughout the research is that of a pluralistic (and segmented) institution in which the meanings of success for each of the constituent groups on each of the criteria of success are contextually determined. That is, they are dependent upon the members' interests, the situation in which they find themselves and the particular tasks that they must accomplish in that setting. The degree to which each group achieves success, as its members define it, then varies with the members' power, their tactics, their acumen and the degree of opposition that they encounter in the gambits of those who construe and pursue the hospital's success in other ways. In drawing together the threads of a pluralistic evaluation we must therefore relate both constituent group interests and performance to success. For as we have argued throughout the study, an account of the social processes through which success is accomplished (or not), in line with group interests, is part and parcel of an evaluative exercise.

Group interests in different patterns of patient flow are especially clear and our account of the hospital's achievements on this count explained how support for 'turnover' in general only yields specific advantages when idiosyncratically interpreted.

We considered consultant interests first. Apart from legal and professional power there are several ways in which consultants can prevent blockage in aspects of the system which are of most concern to them; control bombardment, discharge patients whenever possible, refer patients to other services, and make use of short-term beds. Each of these tactics creates problems for some other groups.

Nursing staff also have strategies for dealing with the 'silt up' in the hospital. They negotiate with relatives their understanding of the terms of admission and they generally favour a rather selective approach to admission. This approach creates some problems for relatives and social work services but the interests of nursing staff and consultant are close in these matters and their combined influence is generally overriding.

GPs' requirements are for facilities which will help them cope with any elderly patients who are making, in their opinion, excessive demands on their time and energy. It is this need which brings them into conflict with day hospital staff, who feel that they must retain selectivity in order to avoid 'silting up' of their part of the system. For ward staff the major interest is in enhancing patient flow out of in-patient wards through the day hospital. That approach generates problems for the day hospital by blocking that part of the system if the patients do not in practice move on.

For the social worker the general principle of the need to maintain patient flow is tempered with concern for the needs of the family unit. In practical terms it is the existence or not of a family capable of looking after the patient that largely determines the nature and possibility of discharge 'to the community'. Because such practical concerns are not uppermost in the work of other staff who see themselves as primarily members of the hospital, a medically oriented view may be rather different from the social work perspective. In this respect therefore the social worker is in an isolated position with interests quite distinctly different in key respects from all other staff groups.

There are also relatives. Although there are exceptions, for the most part they have little interest in or expectation of patient discharge from the day hospital. Much depends upon the way in which the relatives perceive 'the problem' of the patient. Their attitudes towards the patients, the difficulties they face and the hospital's services are largely a function of the way in which they perceive and define the problems with the patients. Frequently this perception of the problem is not in accord with medical and other professional accounts of the patient's difficulties. In consequence, staff perceptions of the advantages of 'turn-over' and the benefits of discharge to patients and relatives, are at cross-purposes with the perceptions of the relatives themselves. In particular, success from the point of view of consultants and nurses is achieved by adopting strategies which militate against the achievement of success as understood by relatives (as well as by other groups of staff).

Another example of the way in which outcomes and notions of success very much depend upon the interests of the groups involved is to be found in our general conclusions about the success of the day hospital in its impact on related services. Difficulties arise in this aspect of the hospital's work because it is not often in the interest of any major group within the day hospital to contribute significantly to an outside service. That is why, we concluded, overall, the day hospital has done little to resolve the long-standing problems in service co-ordination which exist in the field of care for the elderly.

On the criteria of clinical cure and relative support, too, we need no longer labour the point that there are divergent views and different group interests – especially as between staff and relatives. The point of particular relevance to the present discussion is to note why it is that relatives appear to be so limited in their ability to exercise influence. We have said that they do have some tactics through which they may obtain a hospital place for a patient. They do control access to much information about the patient and this they may seek to use for their own purposes. They may form liaisons with staff whom they consider may be able to assist them. Relatives also wield considerable power in their ability to harass the consultant and other staff. This influence is consistently limited, however, by relatives being excluded from any but peripheral roles in the organized services.

This proces is best illustrated in the workings of the relatives' group. Although both staff and relatives benefit from the interaction, in areas of differing interests staff retain clear control.

The culture of success

In summary, we have outlined the performance of the day hospital on each of six criteria of success. We have also shown how group interests interact in the light of what is variously deemed to count as success on each criterion. We have recalled from our findings some illustrations of this process. There is one further step to be taken in the analysis and it stems from an observation that we have made repeatedly throughout this research. Sometimes because of factors external to the hospital and sometimes because of the different constituent interests that we have described, hospital performance, on various counts, variously interpreted, is *not* a success. Many of the points that we have made throughout this report will be read as supporting that conclusion. Yet none of the constituent groups that we have mentioned has a vested interest in the day hospital being seen as a failure. Thus, we have noted, throughout the institution, whatever the performance, whatever the judgements, on whatever criterion, with whatever effect, and on whatever interests, a general 'culture of success' has proved to be remarkably resilient. No matter how each constituent group operationalizes the evaluative criteria, there is common concern, *at an abstract level*, to promote a general ideology portraying the day hospital as a very positive response to the problems of caring for the elderly mentally infirm. We have criticized the presumption of consensus in professional organizations as a basis for evaluating performance in practice. There is, however, a high degree of consensus in promoting the *image* of the day hospital as a success.

Sometimes this is achieved by switching between criteria. We have noted, for example, how a very favourable light may be cast on the hospital's activities by moving between, and sometimes, equating, success as patient flow and success as clinical cure. Similarly success as integrated service and success as impact on related services are sometimes combined and confused in a way which obscures the more obvious deficiencies of interprofessional rivalries and failures to co-operate. Most important of all, success as quality service is used as the 'fall back' position. As we pointed out in our conclusion to Chapter 11, a culture of success is essential to the institution's functioning and the criterion of quality of care serves, if all else fails, to maintain the view that in whatever other ways the hospital might be deficient, in the quality of its attempt it must be rated a success. There is a high level of agreement on this general point and it is exploited throughout the hospital to the full.

On individual criteria, there are also a variety of ways in which the hospital is geared to promoting a successful idelogy. We considered the point at some length, for example, in describing how a 'culture of cure' is maintained. An image of success for the institution as a whole is supported by selective quotation, a set of professional rituals, the use of the notion of 'assessment' to avoid the concept of failure and the variable claim to only limited expertise. Ambiguity and imprecision surrounding the original problem definition also mean that no clear standard exists for demonstrable failures in the treatment regime. In respect of individual cases several practices obfuscate the need to account for failure. Discussion is brief, attention is diverted to success in obtaining a bed for a patient who has deteriorated, the attention of relatives is directed to patients who are in an even worse condition - and so on.

Ritual is *very* important. In discussing the provision of an integrated service, to take another example, we found it hard to avoid the conclusion that much of the collaborative decision-making was apparent rather than real. However, the holding of a regular Tuesday meeting and the mere occurrance of the practices of consultation and decision-making serve actively to foster an image of team activity and allow staff of all grades and specialities to value this as an end in itself. The importance of the meeting, in this context, thus lies in the fact that it maintains what we referred to in passing as the 'myth' of team work, co-ordinated services and thus 'success'.

The existence of the relatives' group is also very important as a ritual. Time and again staff are able to point to the day hospital's commitment to a service to relatives by describing the relatives' group, quite apart from any analysis of how the group actually operates. Indeed, as we showed, although the relatives' group effectively limits the practical implementation of 'relative involvement' to a self-contained and rather isolated locale, thus minimizing the problem of relative disturbance to the organization overall, its mere existence maintains an ideology of service to relatives and thus presents a successful image of the hospital on this criterion.

So, in these several ways, an ideology and culture of achievement is supported and the representation and reputation of success is sustained, even, sometimes at least, in the face of evidence that might be taken to support a contrary view.

Advantages of pluralistic evaluation

We have not attempted in this chapter to summarize in their entirety the detailed materials that we have presented on the workings of the day hospital's services. We have, however, drawn upon our data in order to highlight the major features and key characteristics of a pluralistic evaluation. We have described this approach to evaluative research as solving at least some of the difficulties that we encountered as we embarked on this project and generally it has several very important advantages.

(1) It provides a complicated but realistic answer to the question of whether a service is successful or not. Much research has indicated that most health and welfare institutions fail to live up to their utopian ideals. That is not surprising for, as we have shown, as a matter of ideology, agencies are typically described in highly successful terms. The professional providers and planners of a service are likely to eulogize over a service's performance. Pluralistic evaluation is likely to indicate that in some ways a service is a success and in some ways it is not. As a general comment that is trite. But if we know which aspects of the service are which, that is immensely valuable.

(2) This form of evaluation has the potential to explain *why* 'failures' in service provision occur. Most often this explanation will take the form of an account of which groups have been able to marshal power and resources to pursue their interests, and at what cost to other groups and other forms of service provision. Thus the social processes through which the service fails (by some criteria) are displayed by this form of evaluation, and not merely the service outcomes.

(3) This explanation (as an intrinsic part of the evaluation) opens the way for change. Planners, professionals and adminstrators can see (if they so choose) which groups must be assisted and supported if their objectives and interpretations are to gain effect. Evaluation is limited if it cannot indicate how deficiencies and weaknesses can be rectified.

(4) Pluralistic evaluation details some of the costs of success. Few operational policies are entirely free of unanticipated consequences and it is important to be aware of these consequences even when faced with what is apparently a 'successful' policy in general terms.

(5) Pluralistic evaluation should facilitate the implementation of research results. One major barrier to effective implementation of the policy suggestions of social research has always been opposition from groups who claim that the

research design did not take into account their particular interests. Since pluralistic evaluation cannot be dismissed as dominated by the perspective of a limited group or groups, there would seem to be a greater chance of effective policy implementation based on the research results.
(6) Evaluative studies are often commissioned because the sponsors seek some 'neutral' or 'objective' assessment of the work of an agency. But this is hard to achieve since much evaluation is, implicitly, tied ideologically to a particular perspective on the services. Pluralistic evaluation stands some chance of remaining 'independent' and 'neutral' by taking sympathetic account of as many perspectives as possible.

Some outstanding issues

In conclusion we turn briefly to some issues that are still outstanding in evaluative research for we are far from complacent about the limited progress that has been made in line with suggestions for a new direction in the theory and methodology of evaluation. Some reference, if only brief, to these problems is important because, as we argued in the first chapter of this book, failure to acknowledge some of the implicit difficulties of evaluation has in the past been a cause of considerable confusion.

(1) It may be a mistake to link the methods of pluralistic evaluation to the pluralistic model of policy analysis. The issue is whether it is possible to use pluralistic methods with a 'conflict model' of policy analysis, or indeed with any other framework. Some social commentators would argue that a pluralistic model is by no means universally adequate. We are aware of the major criticisms of pluralism and have referred to some of them in discussing our methods. But if pluralistic evaluation is limited to those institutions and policies of which a pluralistic model is an adequate account, the approach may not be as widely relevant as we have initially implied.
(2) Pluralistic evaluation entails the heavy use of qualitative data. There is a problem in the implementation of policy recommendations that rest upon the interpretation of qualitative results. Although we have explained why pluralistic evaluation has some distinct advantages with respect to implementation, it is clear that both the general approach of the method and, especially, qualitative data are far from the 'scientific' study that many administrators and professionals expect. They may be resistant to them as a result.
(3) Just as there may be a problem of implementing results, so there may be a problem in obtaining the support of administrators and professionals in commissioning pluralistic evaluation.
(4) There is a particular problem of data exclusion in conducting pluralistic evaluation. We have explained how the perspectives of particular constituent groups were defined and their inclusion justified. We also explained that some groups were excluded. The major danger is that in selecting certain groups the investigator adopts a model of the institution and the policy process which is itself biased towards one particular set of interests.

(5) It may be a mistake to view evaluation as a separate kind of social research. We have stressed that adequate evaluation should entail explanation. It has often been argued, equally forcefully, that explanation in social science cannot avoid an evaluative component. If these two arguments converge, then the distinction that is sometimes drawn between evaluative and non-evaluative research may be artificial to a considerable degree.

References

Albrow, M. (1968). 'The Study of Organizations – Objectivity or Bias?' in Gould, J. (ed.) *Penquin Social Science Survey*, Harmondsworth, Penguin.

Allen, I. (1983a). *Short Stay Residential Care for the Elderly*, London, Policy Studies Institute.

Allen, I. et al. (1983b). 'The Elderly and their Informal Carers', in *Elderly People in the Community: Their Service Needs*, London, HMSO, Ch. 5, 69–91.

Asquith, S. (1977). 'Relevance and Lay Participation in Juvenile Justice', *British Journal of Law and Society*, **4**, 61–76.

Austin, N.K. et al. (1976). 'A Comparative Evaluation of Two Day Hospitals', *The Journal of Nervous and Mental Disease*, **163**(4), 253–262.

Baker, A.A. and Byrne, R.J.F. (1977). 'Another Style of Psychogeriatric Service', *British Journal of Psychiatry*, **130**, 123–126.

Barber, J.H. and Wallis, J.B. (1976). 'An information system on the needs of the elderly', *Health Bulletin*, November, **34** (6), 324–330.

Barnes, R.F. et al. (1981). 'Problems of families caring for Alzheimer patients: use of a support group', *Journal of the American Geriatrics Society*, **29** (2), 805.

Bates, T. et al. (1981). 'The St. Thomas' Hospital Terminal Care Support Team', *The Lancet*, May, **30**, 1201–1203.

Becker, H.S. (1958). 'Problems of Inference and Proof in Participant Observation', *American Sociological Review*, **23** (6), 652–660.

Becker, H.S. (1970). *Sociological Work: Method and Substance*, London, Allen Lane, The Penguin Press.

Bell, C. and Newby, H. (eds.) (1977). *Doing Sociological Research*, London, George Allen and Unwin.

Benington, J. (1975). 'The Flaw in the Pluralist Heaven: Changing Strategies in the Coventry CDP', Ch. 19 in Lees R. and Smith G. (eds.) *Action-Research in Community Development*, London, Routledge and Kegan Paul, 174–187.

Benney, M. and Hughes, E.C. (1956). 'Of Sociology and the Interview', American Journal of Sociology **16**, 137–142. Reprinted as Reading 13 in N.K. Denzin (ed.) (1978) *Sociological Methods: A Sourcebook*, New York, McGraw Hill.

Berger, M.M. and Berger, L.F. (1971). 'An Innovative Programme for a Private Psychogeriatric Day Centre', *Journal of the American Geriatrics Society*, **19** (4), 332–336.
Berger, P.L. and Luckmann, T. (1967). *The Social Construction of Reality*, London, Allen Lane, The Penguin Press.
Bergmann, K. et al. (1978). 'Management of the Demented Elderly Patient in the Community', *British Journal of Psychiatry*, **132**, 441–449.
Billis, D. et al. (1980). *Organizing Social Services Departments*, London, Heinemann.
BIOSS (Brunel Institute of Organization and Social Studies) (1974). *Social Services Departments: Developing Patterns of Work and Organization*, London, Heinemann.
Blake, D.H. (1968). 'A Day Hospital for Geriatric Patients: The First Twelve Months', *The Medical Journal of Australia*, November, **2** (18), 802–804.
Blaxter, M. (1976). *The Meaning of Disability: A Sociological Study of Impairment*, London, Heinemann.
Blaxter, M. (ed.) (1979). 'The Analysis of Qualitative Data: A Symposium' *The Sociological Review* (Special Issue), **27** (4).
Brocklehurst, J.C. and Tucker, J.S. (1980). *Progress in Geriatric Care*, London, King Edward's Hospital Fund for London.
Bulmer, M. (ed.) (1977). *Sociolgical Research Methods*, London, Macmillan.
Bulmer, M. (ed.) (1978). *Social Policy Research*, London, Macmillan.
Bulmer, M. (1982). *The Uses of Social Research: Social Investigation in Public Policy Making*, London, George Allen and Unwin.
Caird, F.I. and Judge, T.G. (1979). *Assessment of the Elderly Patient* (2nd edn.), London, Pitman.
Cantley, C. and Smith, G. (1983). 'Social Work and a Relatives' Support Group in a Psychogeriatric Day Hospital: A Research Note', *The British Journal of Social Work*, **13** (6) 663–670.
Carley, M. (1980). *Rational Techniques in Policy Analysis*, London, Heinemann.
Carney, M.W.P. et al. (1970). 'Psychiatric Day Hospital and Community', *Lancet*, **i**, 1218–1220.
Carver, C. and Liddiard, P. (eds.) (1978). *An Ageing Population: A Reader and Sourcebook*, Sevenoaks (Kent), Hodder and Stoughton in Association with the Open University Press.
Charlesworth, A. et al. (1984). *Carers and Services: A Comparison of Men and Women Caring for Dependent Elderly People*, Manchester, Equal Opportunities Commission.
Cherns, A.B. et al. (1972). *Social Science and Government: Policies and Problems*, London, Tavistock.
Cochrane, A.L. (1972). *Effectiveness and Efficiency: Random Reflections on Health Services*, London, The Nuffield Provincial Hospitals Trust.
Copeland, J.R.M. et al. (1975). 'Evaluation of a Psychogeriatric Service: The Distinction Between Psychogeriatric and Geriatric Patients', *British Journal of Psychiatry*, **126**, 21–29.
Cosin, L. (1971). 'Architectural and Functional Planning for a Geriatric Day Hospital', *International Journal of Social Psychiatry*, Spring, **17** (2), 133–140.
Crawford, E. and Perry, N. (1976). *Demand for Social Knowledge: The Role of Research Organizations*, London and Beverley Hills, Sage.
Cronbach, L.J. et al. (1980). *Toward Reform of Program Evaluation*, San Francisco and London, Josey-Bass.
Cross, K.W. et al. (1972). 'Psychiatric Day Care: The New Chronic Population?' *British Journal of Private and Social Medicine*, **26**, 195–204.
Daatland, S.O. (1982). 'Care Systems', *Ageing and Society*, **2** (1), 1–21.
Denzin, N.K. (1978a). *The Research Act in Sociology: A Theoretical Introduction to Sociological Methods* (2nd edn.), New York, McGraw Hill.

Denzin, N.K. (ed.) (1978b). *Sociological Methods: A Sourcebook*, New York, McGraw Hill.

Douglas, J. (1976). *Investigative Social Research: Individual and Team Field Research*, Beverley Hills and London, Sage.

Ellis, L.J. (1974). 'Designing Day Hospitals', *Gerontologica Clinica*, Basel, **16** (516), 294–295.

Eldridge, J.E.T. and Crombie, A.D. (1974). *A Sociology of Organizations*, London, Allen and Unwin.

Erickson, R.C. and Backus, F.I. (1973). 'Symptom severity and day hospital admission', *Hospital and Community Psychiatry*, February, **24** (2), 102–104.

Fennell, G. et al. (1981). *Day Centres for the Elderly in East Anglia*, Norwich, Centre for East Anglian Studies, University of East Anglia.

Fuller, J. et al. (1979). 'Dementia: support groups for relatives', *British Medical Journal*, (1), 1684–1685.

Gandy, John et al. (eds.) (1983). *Improving Social Intervention: Changing Social Policy and Social Work Practice through Research*, London, Croom Helm; New York, St. Martin's Press.

Garland, B. et al. (1981). 'Reevaluating the Place of Evaluation in Planning for Alternatives to Institutional Care for the Elderly', *Journal of Social Issues*, **37** (3), 51–67.

George, V. and Wilding, P. (1976). *Ideology and Social Welfare*, London, Routledge and Kegan Paul.

Gilhooly, M. (1982). 'Social Aspects of Senile Dementia', in Taylor, R. and Gilmore, A. (eds.), *Current Trends in British Gerontology*, Aldershot (Hampshire), Gower, 61–76.

Gilliard, G. and Watt, G. (1982). 'The Impact of Pshchogeriatric Day-Care on the Primary Supporter of the Elderly Mentally Infirm', in Taylor R. and Gilmore, A. (eds.) *Current Trends in British Gerontology*, Aldershot (Hampshire), Gower, 139–147.

Glaser, B.J. and Strauss, A. (1967). *The Disovery of Grounded Theory*, Chicago, Aldine Publishing Company.

Goldberg, E.M. (1984). 'Evaluation Studies: Post Experience and Possible Future Directions', *Research, Policy and Planning*, **2** (1) 1–6.

Goldberg, E.M. et al. (1970). *Helping the Aged: a Field Experiment in Social Work*, London, George Allen and Unwin.

Goldberg, E.M. and Connelly, N. (eds.) (1981). *Evaluative Research in Social Care*, London, Heinemann.

Goldberg, E.M. and Connelly, N. (1982). *The Effectiveness of Social Care for the Elderly*, London, Heinemann.

Goldstein, S. et al. (1968). 'The Establishment of a Psychogeriatric Day Hospital' *Canadian Medical Association Journal*, May 18, **98**, 955–959.

Goldstein, S. et al. (1975). 'The Team Approach in a Psychogeriatric Unit', *Journal of the American Geritrics Society*, **XXIII** (8), 370–375.

Goldstein, S. and Carlson, S. (1976). 'Evaluation of an Active Psychogeriatric Day Hospital', *Canadian Medical Association Journal*, Nov. 6, **115**, 874–876.

Greene, J.G. and Timbury, G.C. (1979). 'A Geriatric Psychiatry Day Hospital Service: A Five-Year Review', *Age and Ageing*, **8** (49), 49–53.

Greene, J.G. et al. (1982). 'Measuring Behavioural Disturbance of Elderly Demented Patients in the Community and its Effects on Relatives: A Factor Analytic Study', *Age and Ageing*, **11**, 121–126.

Grieff, S.A. and McDonald, R.D. (1973). 'Roles of Staff in a Psychogeriatric Day Care Centre', *The Gerontologist*, **13** Spring (1), 39–44.

Hall, P. et al. (1975). *Change, Choice and Conflict in Social Policy*, London, Heinemann.

Hammond, P. (1964). *Sociologists at Work*, New York, Basic Books.

Hardiker, P. (1977). 'Social Work Ideologies in the Probation Service', *The British Journal of Social Work*, 7, 131–154.

Hemsi, L. (1982). 'Living with Dementia', *Postgraduate Medical Journal*, 58, 610–617.
Hildick-Smith, M. (1974). 'Typical Journey to and from Day Hospital', *Gerontologica Clinica*, **16** (5–6) 263–269.
Hill, M. (1983). *Social Policy* (2nd edn.), Oxford, Basil Blackwell and Martin Robertson.
House, E.R. (1980). *Evaluating with Validity*, London and Beverley Hills, Sage.
Hunter, D.J. (1980). *Coping with Uncertainty*, London, Wiley.
Hunter, D.J. and Cantley, C. (1984). 'Exploring Service Variations in the Care of the Elderly: A Voyage into the Interior', in Bromley, D.B. (ed.), *Gerontology: Social and Behaviournal Perspectives*, Beckenham (Kent), Croom Helm.
Hyman, H.H. and Wright, C.R. (1968). 'Evaluating Social Action Programs', Ch. 27 in Lazarsfield, P.F., Sewell, W.H. and Wilensky, H. (eds.), *The Uses of Sociology*, London, Weidenfield and Nicolson, 741–782.
Illsley, R. (1980). *Professional or Public Health?*, London, Nuffield Provincial Hospitals Trust.
Irvine, J. et al. (eds.) (1979). *Demystifying Social Statistics*, London, Pluto Press.
Irvine, R.E. (1969). 'Physiotherapy and the Geriatric Day Hospital', *Physiotherapy*, **55** (9), 352–357.
Isaacs, B. et al. (1972). *Survival of the Unfittest; A Study of Geriatric Patients in Glasgow*, London, Routledge and Kegan Paul.
Isaacs, A.D. and Post, F. (eds.) (1978). *Studies in Geriatric Psychiatry*, Chichester and New York, Wiley.
Johnson, J.M. (1975). *Doing Field Research*, London, Collier-Macmillan.
Jones, I.G. and Munbodh, R. (1982). 'An Evaluation of a Day Hospital for the Demented Elderly', *Health Bulletin* **40** (1), 10–15.
Kanowski, S. (1978). 'The Academic Tasks in Gerontopsychiatry', Ch. 11 in Isaacs, A.D. and Post, F. (eds.), *Studies in Geriatric Psychiatry*, Chichester, Wiley, 219–240.
Kelman, H.R. (1980). 'The Underdevelopment of Evaluative Research on Health Services for the Elderly in the United States', *International Journal of Health Services*, **10** (3), 501–511.
Kinnaird, J. et al. (eds.) (1981). *The Provision of Care for the Elderly*, Edinburgh, Churchill Livingstone.
Knapp, W.S. (1981). 'On the Validity of Accounts About Everyday Life, *The Sociological Review*, **29** (3) 543–562.
Lazarus, L.W. et al. (1981). 'A pilot study of an Alzheimer patients' relatives' discussion group', *Gerontologist*, 21 (4), 353–358.
Levin, E. et al. (1983). *The Supporters of Confused Elderly Persons at Home: Extract from the Main Report*, London, National Institute for Social Work Research Unit (Mimeo).
Lindblom, C.E. (1959). 'The Science of "Muddling Through"', *Public Administration*, **19**, 79–99.
Lofland, J. (1971). *Analyzing Social Settings*, New York, Wadsworth.
McDonald, R.D. et al. (1971). 'Description of a Non-Residential Psychogeriatric Day-Care Facility', *The Gerontologist*, **11** (4), Part 1, Winter, 322–328.
McGrew, A.G. et al. (eds.) (1982) *Decision Making: Approaches and Analysis*, Manchester University Press.
Marsden, C.D. (1978). 'The Diagnosis of Dementia', Ch. 5 in Isaacs, A.D. and Post, F. (eds.), *Studies in Geriatric Psychiatry*, Chichester, Wiley, 95–118.
Martin, A. and Millard, P.H. (1975) 'The The new patient index – a method of measuring the activity of day hospitals', *Age and Ageing*, 4, 119–122.
May, D. (1971). 'Delinquency Control and the Treatment Model: Some Implications of Recent Legislation', *British Journal of Criminology*, **11** (4).
May, D. and Smith, G. (1980). 'Executing Decisions in the Children's Hearings', *Sociology*, **14** (4), 581–601.

Mishra, R. (1981). *Society and Social Policy: Theories and Practices of Welfare* (2nd edn.), London, Macmillan.
Mishra, R. (1984). *The Welfare State in Crisis*, Brighton, Wheatsheaf Books.
Morton, E.V.B. et al. (1968). 'The Joint Assessment and Early Treatment Unit in Psycho-Geriatric Care', *Gerontologica Clinica* **10** (2), 65–73.
Page, S. (1976). 'Towards evaluating the meaningfulness of legal counsel for psychiatric patients', *Canadian Mental Health*, 24 (3), 6–11.
Parlett, M. and Hamilton, D. (1977). 'Evaluation as Illumination: A New Approach to the Study of Innovatory Programmes', in D. Hamilton et al. (eds.), *Beyond the Numbers Game*, London, Macmillan.
Pathy, M.S. (1969). 'Day Hospitals for Geriatric Patients', *The Lancet*, September 6, **2** (619), 533–535.
Peace, S.M. (1980). *Caring from day to day: a Report on the Development of the Day Hospital within the Service for Elderly People who are Mentally Infirm*, Leeds, Mind (Mimeo).
Peach, H. and Pathy, M.S. (1978). 'Social Support and Patients Attending a Geriatric Day Hospital', *Journal of Epidemiology and Community Health*, **32**, 215–218.
Perrow, C. (1963). 'Goals and Power Structures – a Historical Case Study' in E. Freidsen (ed.), *The Hospital in Modern Society*, New York, Free Press.
Phillips, D.L. (1973). *Abandoning Method*, London, Jossey-Bass.
Pitts, J.Y. (1974). 'Psychogeriatric care: A programme for hospital treatment', *Nursing Times*, August 29, **79** (835), 1342–1343.
Platt, S.D. et al. (1980). 'Caution and conservatism in the use of a psychiatric day hospital – Evidence from a research project that failed', *Psychiatry Research*, **3** (2), 123–133.
Rathod, N.H. and Vandrey, B.H. (1971). 'Factors associated with assignment to treatment', *Acta Psychiatrica Scandinavia*, **47** (4), 368–398.
Rein, M. (1976). *Social Science and Public Policy*, Harmondsworth, Penguin.
(1983). *From Policy to Practice*, London, Macmillan.
Robertson, A. and Gandy, J. (1983). 'Policy, Practice and Research: An Overview', Ch. 10 in Gandy, J. et al. *Improving Social Intervention: Changing Social Policy and Social Work Practice Through Research*, London, Croom Helm; New York, St. Martin's Press, 241–289.
Robertson, D. et al. (1977). 'A Community-Based Continuing Care Program for the Elderly Disabled: An Evaluation of Planned Intermittent Hospital Readmission, *Journal of Gerontology*, **32** (3), 334–339.
Ron, M.A. et al. (1979). 'Diagnostic Accuracy in Presenile Dementia', *British Journal of Psychiatry*, **134**, 161–168.
Sanford, J.R.A. (1975). 'Tolerance of Debility in Elderly Dependents by Supporters at Home: Its Significance for Hospital Practice', *British Medical Journal*, (3), 471–473.
Schwartz, M. and Alwin, F. (1971). 'The Evaluation of Social Action', Ch. 21 in Smigel, E.O. (ed.) *Handbook on the Study of Social Problems*, Chicago, Rand McNally, 601–634.
Selltiz, C. et al. (1966). *Research Methods in Social Relations*, London, Methuen.
Sheldon, B. (1984). 'Group-Controlled Experiments in the Evaluation of Social Work Services', in Lishman, J. (ed.) *Evaluation*, Research Highlights 8, University of Aberdeen, 47–67.
Sheldon, F. (1982). 'Supporting the Supporters; Working with the Relatives of Patients with Dementia, *Age and Ageing*, **11**, 184–188.
Shulman, K. and Arie, T. (1978). 'Fall in Admission Rate of Old People to Psychiatric Units', *British Medical Journal*, 21 January, 157–158.
Silverman, D. (1979). *The Theory of Organizations*, London, Heinemann.

Silverman, W.H. and Val, E. (1975) 'Day hospital in the content of a community health programme', *Community Mental Health Journal*, 11, 1, 82–90.
Smith, G. (1979). *Social Work and the Sociology of Organizations* (2nd edn.), London, Routledge and Kegan Paul.
Smith, G. (1980). *Social Need: Policy, Practice and Research*, London, Routledge and Kegan Paul.
Smith, G. and May, D. (1980). 'The Artificial Debate between Rationalist and Incrementalist Models of Decision Making', *Policy and Politics*. 8 (2), 147–161.
Smith, G. and Cantley, C. with Ritman, V. (1983). Patient Turnover in a New Psychogeriatric Day Hospital: a Pluralistic Evaluation', *Ageing and Society*, 3 (3) 325–354.
Stevenson, O. (1983). 'Research on Policy in the Personal Social Services', Ch. 2 in Gandy, J. et al. (eds.) *Improving Social Intervention*, London, Croom Helm; New York, St. Martin's Press, 22–50.
Strauss, A. et al. (1964). *Psychiatric Ideologies and Institutions*, London, Collier-Macmillan.
Taylor-Gooby, P. and Dale, J. (1981). *Social Theory and Social Welfare*, London, Edward Arnold.
Thomas, D. (1982). 'The Terminal Care Support Team', *St Thomas's Hospital Gazette*, 80 (2), 37–39.
Thompson, K. (1980). 'Organizations as Constructors of Reality (1)', Ch. 10 in Salaman, G. and Thompson, K. *Control and Ideology in Organizations*, Milton Keynes, the Open University Press, 216–217.
Tinker, A. (1981). *The Elderly in Modern Society*, Harlow, Essex, Longman.
Voysey, M. (1975). *A Constant Burden: The Reconstitution of Family Life*, London, Routledge and Kegan Paul.
Wadsworth, M.E.J. et al. (1972). 'A Geriatric Day Hospital and its System of Care', *Social Science and Medicine*, **6**, 507–525.
Watts, F.N. and Bennett, D.H. (1978). 'Social Deviance in a Day Hospital', *British Journal of Psychiatry*, **132**, 455–462.
Weale, A. (1983). *Political Theory and Social Policy*, London, Macmillan.
Weiss, C.H. (1972). *Evaluation Research: Methods of Assessing Program Effectiveness*, Englewood Cliffs, New Jersey, Prentice Hall.
Werry, J.S. et al. (1974). 'Evaluating Psychiatric Programmes', *New Zealand Medical Journal*, 23 October, **80** (526), 329–335.
Wheeler, S. (ed.) (1969). *On Record: Files and Dossiers in American Life*, New York, Russell Sage Federation.
Wheatley, V. (1980). *Supporters of Elderly Persons with Dementing Illness Living in the Same Household*, unpublished M.Sc. thesis, University of Surrey.
Whitehead, T. and Mankikar, G. (1974). 'Geriatric Psychiatry in the General Hospital', *The Lancet*, June 15, 1213–1215.
Williams, R.G.A. (1980). 'Innovation in Community Care and General Practice: A Study of Interpretations of a Day Hospital', *Social Science and Medicine*, **14**, 501–510.
Working Group on Terminal Care (1980). 'National Terminal Care Policy', *Journal of the Royal College of General Practitioners*, August, 466–480.
Young, K. and Mills, L. (1978). *Understanding the 'Assumptive Worlds' of Government Actors: Issues and Approaches*, A Report to the SSRC [ESRC] panel on Central Local Government Relations. (Mimeo). School for Advanced Urban Studies, University of Bristol.
Zimmerman, D.H. and Pollner, M. (1971). 'The Everyday World as a Phenomenon', Ch. 4 in Douglas, J.D. (ed.) *Understanding Everyday Life: Towards the Reconstruction of Sociological Knowledge*, London, Routledge and Kegan Paul.

Index